THE SECRET

OF

BIRTH

What every woman should know

about birth and motherhood

REVISED AND UPDATED EDITION

BY KICKI HANSARD

Published by:

CreateSpace Independent Publishing Platform

www.thesecretsofbirth.com

Copyright © Kicki Hansard 2015, 2017.
First edition, November 2015
Revised and updated edition November 2017

ISBN: 978-1517251192

Edited by Jane Hammett
Front and back cover design by Bogdan Stancu
Illustration on front cover and inside book by Annika Langa

Janey Loves Platinum GOLD Award Winner 2017

CONTENTS

For my two beautiful daughters,
Lucy and Cecilia,
who continue to be my greatest teachers,
and for my husband Lance, for his unwavering support

Introduction

Over the past decade, I have encountered hundreds of pregnant women who have all seemed convinced that they needed experts to help them through childbirth and parenting. Often, childbirth is viewed as something medical and highly dangerous, a painful process that seems old-fashioned and outdated. Surely there are better and easier ways to have a baby nowadays? Why would anyone want to have a 'natural' birth?

Initially most women feel excited about being pregnant, although slightly apprehensive – but hopeful that once they have seen a doctor or midwife who will look after them, they will feel better. They book to see a doctor to confirm the pregnancy and come out feeling rather disappointed and even slightly scared. The expectation that someone was going to look after them has not been met and they feel alone; left to figure things out for themselves. The doctor didn't seem quite as excited about the pregnancy as the woman had hoped, and gave no instructions on how they should now continue with their lives as a pregnant woman. What if they do something wrong? What are they actually allowed to do?

Pregnancy somehow makes these intelligent and very capable women feel and believe that they have lost control and knowledge of their body – or perhaps they never had it in the first place? This bothered me a lot, what I was seeing was that women believed that preparing for childbirth and becoming a mother was all outside of themselves. They all felt that they needed someone else to tell them what to do, to be on the safe side, to avoid making a mistake.

Unfortunately, often the only information women have about childbirth is how it is portrayed on the television, on stage or in films. When a woman goes into labour, she clasps her belly and seems to be in intense pain, right from the start. Her waters usually break first. There is usually a lot of blood and a lot of screaming. Even worse, women have watched fly-on-the wall documentaries where birth is portrayed as the worst thing a woman could possibly go through, where film clips have been edited to show a complete lack of support from both partners and hospital staff, and where women in labour are left to fend for themselves. Birth is often shown as the most disempowering event in a woman's life!

I believe that the majority of us are in many ways like these women – unable to distinguish cultural disapproval and media brainwashing from genuine risks when evaluating birth and parenting choices. I started to become frustrated by what I was observing in my clients, as they were intelligent, career-minded women who seemed pretty clear about everything else in their lives. They were all desperately looking for conventional or prescriptive answers, but then often found themselves unable to use that expert knowledge as it often didn't feel right for them.

I have always thought that childbirth should be approached in a completely non-prescriptive way, and that an emphasis on one particular technique or another is a disadvantage to the birthing woman. It is impossible to promote a 'one size fits all' approach that will suit all women. We're all different and live our lives in different ways: some of us are happy-go-lucky and adjust our plans as necessary, while others are more structured and organised, and like to have everything prepared in good time.

We are also hugely influenced by where we grow up, the family values with which we are raised, and the culture into which we are born, not to mention all we experience, and read, and talk to our friends about. I'd rather see women prepare by putting together their very own personal 'toolkit' for labour and birth, full of different theories and approaches, as it is difficult to know beforehand what will be most helpful when labour starts.

I feel that women need to view childbirth (and mothering) in a different light, as powerful, life-changing events and as great opportunities for personal growth. Surely we need to ask ourselves how we have come to focus more on what pram to buy or what car seat to purchase instead of investing time in fully understanding the possible consequences of the way your baby enters this world? I sincerely believe that it's not a conscious choice that leads women to evade taking responsibility for the way they give birth, but rather a lack of information and understanding of the birth process and its impact on both the woman and the baby. I'm convinced that women are capable and intelligent enough to make strong choices about their baby's birth and the way they parent their child – if they knew of the options available to them and the fact that they are allowed to do what they want. However, in my view, women are not always given the information to enable them to make those choices.

As a mother myself and as an experienced doula, I'm certain that the way a woman is made to feel during childbirth has a massive impact on how she feels about herself. This, in turn, has a knock-on effect in all areas of her life. My years of experience of working with women during pregnancy and childbirth have shown me this first-hand, and I have also discovered how incredibly insightful and empowering birth can be. It teaches us about ourselves – we should embrace birth and see it as a momentous event in a woman's life, a powerful and unique opportunity for change. It really doesn't matter how a woman gives birth, as long as she feels fully part of the experience and completely involved in all the decisions made. I don't want birth to continue being the missed opportunity it can be: an opportunity to grow.

I was so certain about this that I decided to go back to university to study Social Science as a mature student, as well as reading hundreds of books on personal growth and childbirth. As a doula course facilitator, I also immersed myself in over one thousand birth stories, written by the women who have trained with me to become doulas themselves. I have also been present at over a hundred births, supporting the birthing woman as well as her partner. Last year, I decided to get more involved with influencing change in maternity services at the Houses of Parliament, highlighting the lack of focus on birth and its impact on women, and – together with my colleagues at Doula UK – instigated a rewrite of a cross-party manifesto. I have contributed to magazine articles and books and have taken part in a TV documentary about doula support. Some people might even view me as an expert and, as the 'expert', I will show you throughout this book that there is only one expert when it comes to you and your baby – and that is you! This book is not about rebelling against experts or the medical system; it's about the fine balance between gathering and evaluating information and continuously checking in with yourself to feel what is right for you. I am not going to give you a single piece of advice about how you should birth or parent your baby. However, I'm hoping to open your eyes to a new way of looking at, and approaching, childbirth and becoming a mother.

What I have experienced as helpful to my clients is a movement away from blindly trusting the voices of the experts and paying more attention to your inner voice, which is full of wisdom and love: reflect on and become totally aware of the pointless aims of perfectionism and over-planning and stop worrying about what other people think. Birth and parenting are not a competition, and I wish that women would stop comparing their choices or judging each other. It's this comparison and the need to make things 'right' or 'wrong' that hugely contribute to the feelings of guilt which so often accompany childbirth and motherhood.

In this book, I will give you the information I give to everyone I work with, so that you can walk your own path to birthing and mothering your baby. I believe that what you learn in this book will show that you already know more than you think you do, and that you can be confident and trust your instincts and have the courage to say 'no' to those who think they know better.

You will notice that throughout the book, I will often talk about 'women' rather than talking to 'you'. This is because I don't want to come across as knowing you or knowing how you think. I don't want there to be any misconceptions that I'm telling you what to do. I'm hoping that, at times, you will recognise yourself as one of these 'women' I speak about – and, when you do, you can feel reassured that you are not alone in feeling or thinking the way you do.

At the end of each chapter, I have added a section called 'Make it real' which lists a number of questions for you to consider. You might decide to discuss these and share your thoughts with your partner, or you may be welcoming your baby on your own. Either way, spending some time considering the information in these sections will help you to think about what you want – and to make clearer choices.

May you feel informed, inspired and supported by what you read, and may your choices for yourself and your baby benefit from a firm and gentle foundation, based on love as well as instinct. By the time you've finished reading this book, I hope that you will know beyond a shadow of a doubt that you have within yourself everything you need to birth and parent your baby – and that you will be looking forward to the unique experience of giving birth and becoming a mother!

Secret #1

You are allowed to choose, and do, whatever you want!

CR✿SO

Chapter 1: Preparing for Birth

I believe that every pregnant woman is walking around in a light state of hypnosis. Because of this, they are very susceptible to anything they hear or see related to pregnancy and childbirth. In society today, the press and media often paint a very negative picture of childbirth, and women are led to assume that having a baby is somehow impossible without some kind of medical intervention. Childbirth in films or TV dramas is always portrayed in dramatic scenes of crisis, fear and tension. The media seem to consistently portray childbirth as a horrendous and frightening process that anyone in their right mind would want to avoid. It is more or less impossible to get away from all the negativity. Simply taking a bus journey when you are pregnant will often attract someone who is eager to tell a scary story about how somebody they knew nearly died giving birth. Your friends, family and neighbours will also have similar stories which they are keen to tell.

There is also such an overwhelming amount of information about pregnancy and childbirth out there. So many books have been written on how to achieve a pain-free, quick and 'perfect' birth, all focusing on a certain way or technique. Women are led to believe that preparing and planning for the birth in great detail will somehow give them control over what happens. I feel that this need for control is because women are fearful of something not being 'right' or that something will go horribly wrong. However, what many people don't know is that physiological childbirth involves the primitive part of the brain, where all the hormones and endorphins are produced, not the intelligent brain, where the need to control and plan resides. Women should focus on finding a way of keeping their intelligent brain quiet and trusting their body to know what to do. This process happens naturally if the circumstances are right. Surprisingly, for many, the factor that has the biggest impact on childbirth is the environment in which the woman chooses to welcome her baby: it has to be somewhere she feels safe. She also needs to be able to switch off her thinking brain, which might mean she will be acting out of character. The woman might make strange noises, start swearing or screaming and shouting. This is discussed in more detail in Chapter 2.

In order to create a sense of 'being in control', it has become very popular for couples to write a birth plan. They spend hours putting down on paper how the birth should be, with some birth plans running into several pages. I have never been an enthusiastic promoter of birth plans: my belief is that whenever you make a 'plan' you need to have a backup plan and, when it comes to childbirth, you are very likely to need a number of plans. The big flaw with making a 'plan' for childbirth is that this assumes that you have control over what is going to happen and how everyone involved is going to behave, including the baby. It also makes it look as though it is possible to evaluate risk in a logical manner and simply choose one thing over another, to minimise the need for intervention or an unwelcome medicalised birth.

Unfortunately, it's not that simple. There is always a baby involved in the birth process, who is very difficult – if not impossible – to control, and there are a number of things that could happen when labour starts that means the first thing on your birth plan goes out the window. For example, a woman might write that she is planning to stay at home as long as she feels comfortable and happy. However, her waters might break one morning and she might have no contractions for the next twenty-four hours. In this case, she will be advised by her medical care providers, who are following clinical guidelines, to come to hospital for labour to be induced. The reason for this is that there is a misconception that the risk of infection for the baby increases after a woman's waters have broken. However, there is currently no research evidence to support this. There is, however, research to suggest that there is a slight increase in the chance of uterine infection for mothers who wait for labour to start naturally (Dare et al., 2017). Imagine for a minute how this would make her feel. I'm not suggesting that she has to take her care providers' advice; she doesn't. But a spanner has been thrown in the works, so to speak. If this woman had no birth plan in the first place, she might find it easier to accept that it's still possible for her to have the birth she would like – although she may have to slightly adapt it, according to her new circumstances. With a preconceived plan, she might start feeling that everything is going to go wrong, with the result that her mind becomes full of negative thoughts and her body full of stress hormones – not the best way to prepare for birth.

However, I agree that it is a good idea to write something down with regard to your upcoming birth, and I would like to refer to it as *birth preferences* rather than a birth plan. This should consist of no more than one page, containing information about your preferences for pain management and any options for the baby, such as:

- delayed cord clamping (McDonald et al., 2013)
- the administration of vitamin K to the newborn (Wickham, 2001)
- immediate skin-to-skin contact.

The enormous benefits of skin-to-skin are often not known to new parents, and it is therefore often overlooked, as it seems such a small thing, but a Cochrane Review concluded that:

> Babies exposed to skin-to-skin contact interacted more with their mothers and cried less than babies receiving usual hospital care. Mothers were more likely to breastfeed in the first one to four months, and tended to breastfeed longer, if they had early

skin-to-skin contact with their babies. Babies were possibly more likely to have a good early relationship with their mothers, but this was difficult to measure. (Moore et al., 2012)

In my view, there is little point in writing about how you would like a Caesarean birth to be carried out, unless you are planning to have an elective Caesarean. An elective Caesarean is a pre-planned Caesarean due to a medical condition or risk. It is also when a woman makes the choice to give birth via Caesarean, even though there might be no medical reasons to do so. A woman might choose this option for a number of reasons, but often I feel it is because they have not been given enough information about the risks associated with a Caesarean birth or the benefits for both the baby and mother of giving birth vaginally. However, I think every woman has the right to choose for herself how she gives birth.

Caesarean births are a normal way to welcome a baby these days: national statistics in the UK shows that as many as one in four women will give birth this way. If your preference is for a physiological birth, which I will define in the next chapter, there is no need to focus on how to have a Caesarean birth, and if your baby is born by Caesarean in the end, it should be done for good and justifiable reasons. Also, all the things that are important immediately after birth, such as delayed cord clamping and skin-to-skin, should still be facilitated after a Caesarean birth. Spending hours writing birth plans really isn't the best way to prepare for the birth of a baby. Instead, emphasis should be placed on learning about birth hormones, how these are released, and how to create a safe space to welcome your baby.

I'm convinced that if parents-to-be feel they are well informed about their options, they understand the consequences of their choices and they have written down some birth preferences, they are in a much stronger position to have a positive birth experience. My invitation after this is to completely surrender to the birth process – and when I say 'surrender', I don't mean the type of surrendering when you don't care any more and just give up. I'm talking about becoming open and accepting what unfolds in the moment, instead of fighting against it.

Buying the perfect birth experience

Birthing a baby is an outstanding experience in a woman's life, during which she will become aware of some of her vulnerability – but also her incredible power. Giving birth can dramatically change her perception of herself and her self-esteem: most of the time, giving birth has a positive impact.

The birth process generally shapes a woman's experience of motherhood, and will have an effect on how she starts out in her new role as a mother. It's therefore a good idea to carefully consider and explore the different options available when planning for your baby's birth. If you can make strong, informed decisions based on unbiased information which enable you to take responsibility for your birth, you will start from a place of personal power and this will make you feel more in control. There is not one 'correct' way of giving birth, and it's not something that a woman 'fails' or 'passes'. As long as *she* decides what is best for her and her baby, it can be an empowering experience.

During midwife appointments, you will be able to discuss the local options available to you, and it's also a good idea to do some research of your own as well. It is important to have a look at which maternity units are close enough to be considered, and you can also visit them to have a look at the facilities. Each National Health Service (NHS) trust will have clinical guidelines, written to show how they wish care to be provided within maternity services, and these might differ from trust to trust. These guidelines are there to 'guide care', not to dictate how and what must happen. It's very important to remember that the choice of where to give birth is entirely yours, and you can change your mind at any time. A woman can decide to stay at home to give birth if that's what she chooses to do, and the local NHS trust is obliged to provide her with a midwife.

In the UK we have a very good NHS system which provides free maternity services, with many wonderful midwives and doctors. The system is perhaps overstretched in certain areas, which is widely reported in the press, and can lead couples to look into hiring private maternity care.

A question worth contemplating is whether a couple will have a perfect birth experience if they hire their own obstetrician and book a place in a private maternity unit. Imagine the following scenario:

A woman discovers that she is pregnant. Her friends all tell her to first and foremost book an obstetrician, as the most popular ones get booked up very quickly. She is in a position, financially, to do so and she is determined to get the best care money can buy. She is delighted to find that the private hospital she has set her heart on has availability, and also the obstetrician she has heard so many good things about is free. She is delighted and relieved that she can now relax and enjoy her pregnancy, believing that she will receive the best care and up-to-date services available.

Next, she decides to start going to yoga classes and antenatal classes, and she starts reading books about childbirth. She begins to like the idea of a natural birth with the minimum use of drugs. She starts to feel confident in her own body, and wants to take responsibility for her own birth experience. She realises there is research to suggest a link between drugs used in childbirth and drug abuse in later life (Jacobson et al., 1990). She learns that keeping the umbilical cord attached until it stops pulsating, then cutting it, will increase neonatal iron storage at birth (McDonald et al., 2013). She reads that if she has a straightforward natural birth, there is no need to have an injection to deliver the placenta; her body can do this all on its own.

Perhaps she may even decide to hire a doula, as she has learnt that: 'women who received continuous labour support were more likely to give birth 'spontaneously', i.e. give birth with neither Caesarean nor vacuum nor forceps. In addition, women were less likely to use pain medications, were more likely to be satisfied, and had slightly shorter labours' (Hodnett et al., 2017). A doula is a lay person, usually a woman, who provides emotional and practical support, before, during and after childbirth.

She is now feeling happy and excited because she knows so much more about her options and choices; she feels 'in control'. She decides to speak to her obstetrician about her wishes, but during the meeting she finds that they have little common ground. The obstetrician does not share her enthusiasm about birthing the placenta without the use of drugs (or, in medical terms, a physiological third stage), and suggests that she has been fed unrealistic information. The woman starts to feel confused and unsure. She tries to make sense of the situation: surely she is paying this person to give her what *she* wants? The very least she expects is for her obstetrician to listen to her views, discuss them with her and provide reasons – backed up by facts and figures – why he doesn't share her thoughts. She no longer feels happy with any information he gives her that is followed by 'in my view' or 'based on my many years' experience'. The discussion soon moves away from her ideas and birth preferences to talk about induction dates and pain management, and the possible risks due to the size of the baby or its position. The woman starts to get a horrible feeling that her obstetrician wants to schedule her in for an induction two weeks before her due date, even though there is no medical reason for this. She feels growing mistrust and suspicion.

When she leaves the meeting, she feels that communications have broken down and she doesn't feel like speaking to her obstetrician any more. She finds that she starts to keep information from him, and that she dreads each weekly meeting, where she feels unheard and bullied. She starts to worry about what is going to happen when she goes into labour. How can she trust this person to support her in her wishes, and not look for any excuse to go down a medical birth route?

Fortunately, this scenario does not happen all the time, but it does occur more often than you can imagine. I am not suggesting that all obstetricians are nasty, 'out to get you' people who only care about when they can clock off, but I am talking about a very common misconception. Going private does not guarantee that the care you will receive is necessarily the care that you and your partner are looking for. The misconception is what someone means when the say the 'best care'. To a woman, this might mean a comforting voice or hand; someone who will listen to her and be empathetic; someone who will do everything to fulfil her wishes, as long as there are no medical indications to do otherwise. However, to someone else it might mean being able to take advantage of the latest technology; having rigid procedures and protocols in place; preventative medicine; keeping 'on top' of things; removing or actively managing any pain; and trusting the experts. What many people are not aware of is that women who choose to give birth in a private hospital are at an increased chance of a having a surgical birth rather than a normal vaginal birth (Dahlen et al., 2012).

If a woman's choice is to have an elective Caesarean, or she wants an epidural as soon as labour starts, then going down the private route will probably be a good option for her as the NHS isn't always able to accommodate this. In all likelihood, this woman will have made an informed choice and will understand the risks and possible complications associated with these options. A good birth experience is about having made informed choices, about feeling included in any decision-making, and believing that all procedures have been explained in detail. Whether a woman has a drug-free vaginal birth or an elective Caesarean birth is up to her, but it is worth reading up on the pros and cons of each choice. This is a great article to read to gain more information: https://www.bellybelly.com.au/birth/caesarean-section-or-vaginal-birth/

If a woman is looking for a more natural birth with minimum interventions, the best route is to book a home birth. Home births always provide the support of not one, but two, midwives, who trust that the overwhelming majority of women in their care will be able to birth naturally. They will do everything to support a woman to give birth at home, as long as she and the baby are well. Being at home, in a familiar environment, helps women to relax and produce the hormones needed for a straightforward birth. The latest NICE (National Institute for Health and Care Excellence) guidelines recommend that women whose pregnancies are low-risk should consider birthing at home, as it is a very safe option.

If a woman does not want a home birth, the next best place to give birth is in a birth centre or midwife-led unit. This doesn't mean that the woman will have to give birth without pain management. There are pain medication options available both for home and birth centre births, and women can request a transfer to the obstetric unit at any time. Every woman has the right to give birth wherever she chooses to, and she can look at more than one hospital local to her. Remember, a woman is 'allowed' to do what she wants. It is her body, her baby and her birth experience!

If you find the option of hiring a private obstetrician the most appealing, it's worth making sure you find out about their views and philosophy on childbirth. Perhaps look at their rate of Caesarean versus vaginal births. Speak to some of their previous clients, and ask them to be honest about the care they received. When visiting a private maternity unit, find out from the staff what kind of births are most common and, in their view, what kind of priorities the women who come there have. Are they keen to have physiological births or are they looking for the latest technology and pain management? Most midwives will be able to tell a woman whether the place is suitable for her or not, if they know how she sees her ideal birth experience.

A large cohort study was carried out in England called the Birthplace in England Research Programme (Birthplace in England Collaborative Group, 2011). The Birthplace study found that many more women had a 'normal' birth with low levels of intervention if they had their baby somewhere other than a hospital labour ward.

The following overall normal birth rates for all mothers who were low-risk at the start of labour demonstrate this:

- 58% – planned births in an obstetric unit
- 76% – planned births at a birth centre attached to a hospital
- 83% – planned births at a standalone birth centre
- 88% – planned births at home.

These women were all low-risk, which mean they had no complications in their pregnancy and were all healthy, yet when they turned up at an obstetric unit, their chances of having a 'normal' birth were only 58%. In other words, they had a 42% risk of having some form of intervention simply because of where they gave birth. These statistics clearly show that where a woman chooses to give birth heavily influences what kind of a birth experience she will have.

As I said earlier, the birth process is unpredictable, and there is no way to guarantee a perfect birth experience by any means. Each couple needs to work from their own life experiences and personalities, manage their expectations, and understand their rights and choices: after all, each birth is unique.

Antenatal classes
Few NHS trusts now offer free antenatal classes for couples, and the classes that still run, in my opinion, offer limited information. Any antenatal preparation run by a hospital trust will follow the trust's policies and clinical guidelines, so the information provided could be rather one-sided. Even though birth physiology should be the most important item on the list of subjects to cover, I strongly feel that not enough emphasis is put on this. These classes usually cover interventions during birth, pain management options, and what to expect and what to do when labour starts.

They are usually run by an experienced midwife, which is great, but I feel that there might be one vital process missing for many midwives. If they had a birth experience which was not as they had hoped for, or they struggled with breastfeeding, there often isn't the opportunity to debrief this during their training. This could have an impact on how and what they teach, and any deep-held disappointment about what happened to *them* might come across in the sessions. This is true for anyone who teaches antenatal classes. Throwaway comments made by an authority figure or 'expert' can have a huge impact on the women in these classes. Passing a set of forceps or an epidural needle around a class of pregnant women as they prepare to give birth is not helpful, and can be extremely scary. I guess that such gestures are well-meant, as midwives want women to feel fully informed, but there is a fine line between sharing information and creating fear.

Private antenatal classes are usually only as good as the facilitator of the course, and some classes run by the UK's largest charity for parents, the

National Childbirth Trust (NCT), can sometimes feel a bit like preparing for battle with the medical care providers. The NCT has done so much for pregnant and birthing women in the UK, but I think the charity has become too focused on the academic side of birth, often leaving out, or forgetting about, birth physiology. Many classes begin with a catch-up on the previous week, when each couple tell the rest of the group how their week has been. Some people I have spoken to find this boring, and, if there is a woman in the group who is having a difficult pregnancy, it can be hard for the rest of the group to hear about everything that could go wrong. In these classes, couples who are planning home births are often held in slightly higher esteem than couples who are thinking of using pain medication and unsure whether or not to breastfeed. I'm making a very sweeping generalisation here, I realise, but this is what I often hear from the couples I've worked with who have done NCT classes (which is the majority of them). I'd like to point out that there are some excellent NCT teachers out there who do a wonderful job of preparing couples for their upcoming birth and postnatal period. The biggest advantage that many people say they get from antenatal classes is meeting other couples in their area who are also having babies at the same time. This support network is invaluable in the first weeks, months and years as a mother.

I think it is important to do some antenatal birth preparation, and I know that meeting other parents-to-be is crucial. It is especially helpful in the postnatal period to have some friends who are experiencing the same things. Peer support is invaluable, and can make a new and unfamiliar situation become normalised, as the woman is not alone in her experience.

However, I believe very strongly that the purpose of an antenatal class should be to clearly explain that childbirth is a physiological process, so that women and their partners understand that you don't have to study for birth – it just happens! It is, of course, also important to understand the path to birth, the different 'stages' of labour, the pain management options and the impact these can have on the birth process.

What I think is even more important is to learn the positive benefits of having skin-to-skin contact with your newborn, the risks of not breastfeeding, and the huge benefits to the baby of delayed cord clamping. Ultimately, when a woman or couple have finished their antenatal preparation, they should be open to the fact that anything could happen during labour, and they can still have a good birth experience even if things don't go entirely to plan. Antenatal sessions should encourage women and couples to avoid making firm plans, and instead help them focus on writing down what they would like to happen: that is, birth preferences. It is important to trust the birth process and believe that these preferences can be achieved and, at the same time, respect that the process also is uncontrollable.

MAKE IT REAL

You may like to think about, or discuss with your birth partner, the following.

Your birth preferences: Is there anything you would like more information about? You may want to consider your preferences in case your birth takes a different path, so that if medical interventions become necessary, you will feel well prepared and well informed in advance.

Where you would like to give birth: What are your options? Where will you feel most relaxed? As you know, you do not have to decide now, and you can change your mind right up until labour starts. You may wish to research the Birthplace Cohort Study (see www.npeu.ox.ac.uk/birthplace/results) a bit more.

Who you would like to attend the birth: Would you like to hire a doula? Have your mother present? Perhaps you would prefer a private obstetrician? How might having that person or those people at the birth change the dynamic?

Your antenatal preparation: Are you interested in private classes? How will you ensure you are well informed before your baby's birth?

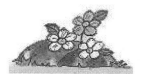

Secret #2

Childbirth

is a

physiological

event

— it just

happens!

CRQEO

Chapter 2: Physiological Childbirth

When I talk about childbirth, I like to refer to it as 'physiological', rather than a 'normal' or a 'vaginal' birth. The reason for this is that a 'normal' birth nowadays could mean a Caesarean birth, since at least one out of four women in the UK will give birth this way. A 'vaginal' birth does not always mean a birth without interventions. The NHS collects data on what constitutes a 'normal' birth, and this simply means that the baby came out of a woman's vagina, even if the birth involved the use of drugs for pain management and the use of instruments (forceps, ventouse) to help the baby be born. Most doulas and midwives talk about a straightforward physiological birth when we are referring to a birth that happened just as nature intended it to happen.

The other trouble with calling something 'normal' means that any other way of giving birth becomes 'abnormal', and for a woman who has an unwanted Caesarean birth, this could add to any feelings of failure she might already have. It's not always what is openly said that is hurtful, but connotations that may be hidden in the language we use can also cause upset.

What does the term 'physiological birth' actually mean?

A physiological process is something that happens in a woman's body with the help of hormones and without her having to engage the 'thinking' brain (or what is also known as the neocortex). Birth is a very normal, physiological body function, and the body knows how to birth. Just as the body knows how to cough, sneeze, produce waste, digest and process foods into energy, so a woman's body knows how to grow and give birth to a baby. Women have been giving birth for many years – some people estimate close to one million years – and the same process that occurs today was happening a thousand years ago in exactly the same way.

We have by no means perfected birth, although birth is generally safer today because of the medical knowledge and technology now available to us. Unfortunately, what we seem to (unintentionally) have done is become less dependent on our body's own ability and more focused on studying and learning how to do childbirth the 'right way'.

The process has become too academic and theory-driven, rather than natural and instinctive. More and more women are under the impression that they can somehow control childbirth by revising, spending time before the birth learning techniques and focusing the majority of their time on preparing for birth in their neocortex. When all the responsibility for the birth outcome is seen as being the result of how well you read up on it, who is to 'blame' if the birth isn't exactly as the woman thought it was going to be? The woman herself, of course – she didn't study well enough! And how is this going to make her feel in the postnatal period? Most likely, she will feel that she is failing or not being a very good mum, as she didn't have the birth she had planned for, so how can she get anything else right?

As birth is physiological and takes place in the old brain (the primitive part) where instinct and hormone release takes place, women should prepare for birth by switching off their thinking brain. They should spend time connecting with their baby in the womb and connecting with their physical body, by doing yoga or some other form of physical exercise.

The only information I think a woman needs to have before giving birth is a complete understanding of birth physiology, so that she knows what she can do to help herself have a straightforward physiological birth.

I'd like to compare it to another physiological process: going to sleep. I'm sure we have all experienced needing to get up early the next morning to catch a flight or go to an important event. We're lying in bed, thinking, 'I need to go to sleep or I'm going to be so tired tomorrow.' The more we try to make ourselves go to sleep, the harder it seems. If instead we think, 'Oh, it doesn't matter if I sleep or not, as long as I rest, I will be fine,' sleep will soon descend upon us. By changing our thinking, we 'trick' our thinking brain and our primitive brain can start producing the hormones we need to go to sleep. Childbirth is pretty much the same.

What happens in a woman's body as she gives birth?
As the baby is getting to the point when it is ready to be born, it will send a signal to the mother's brain to let her know that the time has come. One theory is that it is a protein that brings about the contractions which start labour (Parkington et al., 2014). Another suggestion is that once the baby's lungs have reached maturity, a chemical signal is given to the mother (Mendelson, 2009). However, something triggers the pituitary gland in the woman's brain to start producing the hormone oxytocin. Oxytocin is also known as the 'love hormone', and women have very high levels of oxytocin in their body during labour and breastfeeding as well as during lovemaking.

Oxytocin, the hormone of closeness, is triggered by touch, massage, warmth and love. This hormone is also responsible for the contractions (or, as I prefer to call them, the tightenings) of the uterine muscles that push the baby downwards and pull the cervix open. Oxytocin means 'quick birth' in Greek; the higher the levels of oxytocin in a woman's body, the quicker her birth will be. At the same time as oxytocin is released, the brain will also start producing endorphins. Endorphins are the body's own pain management system, and the word 'endorphin' actually means 'the morphine within' in Greek. The body's endorphins are eighty times more powerful than synthetically produced morphine,

23

and as they are naturally produced, they have no harmful effects on the mother or baby.

Early on in labour, the cervix needs to move from a posterior position (backward-facing) to an anterior position (forward-facing) and then it will start to thin out (or efface, as it is known in medical terms). A woman's cervix feels a bit like the tip of the nose and is made up of a ring muscle (or a sphincter muscle). All sphincter muscles in the body are connected, which means the mouth and the cervix have a correlational relationship. Ina May Gaskin, a world-famous midwife, coined the phrase 'sphincter law' and, according to her observations, the cervix, the vagina, the anus and the urethra open best in an private and intimate environment. She also noted that sphincters open more easily if a woman is laughing or if she is being praised and encouraged, but can also suddenly close if a woman becomes frightened or self-conscious (Gaskin, 2004). I often see women who are choosing to labour in water instinctively put their lips on the surface of the water and snort like a horse, making their lips vibrate, creating bubbles in the water. This is exactly how the cervix should be – relaxed, like soft set jelly, thinning out and expanding over the baby's head.

When labour starts, most women will say they experience tightenings, similar to period pains, in the lower abdomen. The tightenings might come every half an hour, and will gradually increase in length and become closer together. These tightenings are the uterine muscles pulling and pushing, extending and contracting, just like in any other physical event when muscles are involved. It is not a sign that something is wrong, and a baby does not usually become 'distressed' by these tightenings. For the baby, it must feel like being hugged by the uterus, so it probably feels quite nice!

As labour progresses and the cervix is opening, the baby starts to move down through the woman's pelvis. Hormones released during pregnancy will have softened the ligaments and joints and as the baby moves down, some women will feel this in their lower back. It also depends on what position the baby is in, as she is navigating the bony pelvis and finding the best fit, so to speak. Studies show that babies move all the time in labour, and the majority of babies, who may not be in an ideal position at the start of labour, end up in the perfect position for birth. If a woman is left to get in a position in which she is comfortable, it usually is the absolute best position both for her and for her baby. It is also very likely to help the baby turn into an ideal position!

Oxytocin levels and endorphin levels increase quickly when the woman is feeling well supported, the room she is labouring in is warm, and the lights are dimmed. This means that the strong sensations from her uterine muscles working hard are manageable. The woman might experience intense sensations during these tightenings and, by using her breathing and making the most of the breaks in between the tightenings to rest, she will be coping and managing the sensations well. Just like someone climbing a steep hill, running a marathon or lifting weights in a gym, her muscles are working hard. Labour will usually get a bit intense and even painful at times, but thanks to the birth hormones, women are able to cope with that and continue working through it.

Just before – and as – the cervix thins enough to allow the baby's head to come through, like the neck of a polo-neck jumper, women will usually experience tightenings very close together, and this can be a very intense time of labour. As the birth of the baby gets nearer, women will often feel that they can't cope any longer and that they want to go home and not do this any more!

As I said earlier, women have been giving birth for up to a million years, and evolution has not caught up with our changing lifestyle. When we were hunter-gatherers, it was important for us to know that we were in labour, and also very important to know that the baby would be born soon. We are all familiar with the hormone adrenaline, which is released when we feel under threat or stressed. It triggers what is called the 'fight or flight' reflex, where we need to assess the environment we are in and decide whether to stay ('fight') or flee for our lives ('flight'). If we were out collecting food and in early labour as a hunter-gatherer, and felt an adrenaline rush, it would be important for us to start making our way back home. If labour was at the point where the baby could be born, we would need to be back in our cave to give birth in a safe environment for both us and the baby.

This process can still be observed in women today during childbirth. As most women come to the phase in labour that is called *active labour*, which usually means the cervix is opened to around four or five centimetres, there is a release of adrenaline to alert them that they should start making their way back to their 'cave'. This adrenaline triggers the 'fight or flight' reflex, which usually translates into a feeling of fearfulness. As a woman starts feeling fearful in labour, her oxytocin and endorphin levels fall slightly. Because of this, the tightenings of the uterus can feel more intense. As the intensity grows, the woman can become scared and might even start doubting her body's ability to give birth. If she gets increasingly scared, she is likely to enter what is known as the *pain–fear cycle*. The more pain she experiences, the more fearful she gets, which means more adrenaline is released and fewer endorphins, which means more pain. Many women, if in hospital, will often have some type of pain management at this point, even though this adrenaline rush is a primitive warning system, telling women to start making their way to a safe place. This phase usually only lasts for around forty minutes, and as a woman moves into active labour, her oxytocin and endorphins levels will build up again. Being aware that this feeling does not mean something is wrong, but instead actually means things are going well, might be helpful, as many women can interpret this moment in labour as something being wrong. If women knew about the natural rise and fall of the body's hormones during childbirth, it would all make more sense to them and they would not become trapped in the pain–fear cycle.

Again, during the last part of the first stage of labour, adrenaline is released in the body to tell the hunter-gatherer woman that she must get to her cave *now*! That is why many women tend to open their eyes, feel scared and even try to get off the bed to go home during this final stage of the cervix opening up. Women who have been totally focused inwardly, simply breathing, making deep sighing sounds and swaying with the tightenings will become more vocal and look for reassurance from their support team. Many women are familiar with this stage in labour, and it is commonly called *transition* – the transition from the first stage to the second stage of labour.

When the cervix is fully open, the baby can start making her way out through the birth canal. The tightening and releasing of the uterus muscles starts to change, and women usually feel a strong need to push. Many women welcome this feeling, as it's no longer about sinking into the sensations but, at last, working with them. As the baby moves down the birth canal, the need to push increases. Some women worry about pushing too hard: the majority of women worry about their perineum being damaged, or fear they will have a bowel movement at this point. Thinking like this might prevent them from following their bodies' signals and allowing their baby to be born.

Having a bowel movement is a great sign that the baby is coming, and most midwives and doulas get very excited when this happens. Midwives are usually very quick and discreet, and will remove any small bowel movement before anyone has even realised what has happened.

Perineal tears are common in childbirth, and the majority of women will not realise that this has happened until after the baby has been born and the midwife tells her. It is unusual for a woman to actually feel the tearing – and once her baby has arrived, she will be so busy falling in love that it won't feel like a major deal. It is usually a much bigger worry for women as they approach birth, but it is worth bearing in mind that being fearful of tearing or bowel movements could make the second stage of labour longer than it needs to be.

When a baby is born, she will have a sense of smell thirty times more powerful than at any other time in her life! By letting her be born onto her mother's bare skin, she will pick up her mother's natural smell, the baby's intestine will be colonised by the microbiomes from the mother, and the baby will start her life in the best possible way. Keeping mother and baby together and warm for the first hour after birth should be a priority for all involved in the birth.

What does labour feel like?

What most women want to know as they prepare for labour is what it's going to feel like. How painful will it be? Many women have heard so many scary stories and been influenced by the portrayal of births in films and in television programmes that they are often already full of adrenaline and fear. As labour starts, they are unable to focus on what they are actually feeling and experiencing; instead they are worrying about what will happen next. It's like that feeling you might have when you're watching a scary film and you're just waiting for something scary to happen. Having a high level of adrenaline in your body makes your body be on constant 'red alert', and your hearing, sense of smell and readiness for action are all enhanced. If someone grabbed you at this point, you will most likely be very quick to react, probably by screaming and perhaps even hitting out. Your heart will be pounding and all your senses will be over-sensitised. This is very similar to what it's like to approach childbirth full of fear and full of adrenaline.

Birth is actually all in the head: once a woman has got into the right frame of mind, her body will simply follow. A woman full of adrenaline will experience the contractions of the uterine muscles as unbearable, and painful to the point where they become unmanageable. It has nothing to do with 'pain thresholds' or about being tough. It's got everything to do with the woman's personality traits, previous life experiences, her ability to approach the unknown with confidence, and the way she thinks and talks about birthing.

Physiological labour uses hormones to guide the woman and take her to a place which many women refer to as 'planet birth'. Oxytocin is released in waves, and endorphins with it, making her feel as if she is 'out of her body', but still very much present in a way she has probably never experienced before. As her muscles contract and pull, she may feel like a boat at sea, being thrown back and forth, and then having peace and space to recover in the breaks between tightenings. It often makes me think of the film *The Truman Show* when the main character, played by Jim Carrey, tries to escape, and the director of the TV programme creates a storm on the ocean to stop him. But Jim Carrey's character perseveres and battles on until he finally reaches the shore on the other side. He is determined and he knows he's going to make it, as long as he can stay focused on what is happening in the present. Labour and childbirth are very much the same.

The uterus (womb) is one giant muscle that does all the work during childbirth. The oxytocin released from the pituitary gland gets the various muscles to contract and release during labour, and three different layers work in harmony with each other. The inner layer of the uterus consists of circular fibres that go all the way around the uterus. During labour, these muscles relax so that the outer layer can gently nudge the uterus upwards, which opens up the cervix, which is at the bottom of the womb. Once the cervix is fully opened, the outer layer's muscular motion changes and begins to push the baby downwards, during the second stage of labour. There is also a middle layer of muscles in the uterus that allows the free flow of blood to and from the baby. When these middle muscles are contracted, blood supply to the baby is slightly lower than when they are nice and relaxed. It is, therefore, very important that there are breaks in between contractions in labour so that the baby constantly gets a good supply of oxygenated blood. The uterus itself also needs to have a break to get ready for the next round of tightenings. So the muscles of the uterus work in harmony to open the cervix, move the baby downwards and finally expel the baby. It is worth considering that the cervix itself is totally inactive in labour; however, this is what doctors measure and observe. It is the muscles of the uterus that pull the cervix open, and not the cervix itself that opens up. We could, therefore, ask *why* the cervix is what medical professionals measure to assess the progress of labour? All it is actually telling us is what is happening right now, at this point in labour, and not how things will progress. As with everything else in labour, women can decline vaginal examinations.

Interestingly, the inner layer of circular muscles is directly linked to a woman's autonomic nervous system; that is, the survival parts of her brain. If she is getting messages from the environment around her that it is not safe to birth her baby, these muscles will start to contract, instead of release, during the first stage of labour, making the early part of labour (the latent phase) more painful, and usually longer, as the body is fighting itself. Again, the importance of a calming environment for a labouring woman cannot be emphasised enough.

If a woman is willing to accept that the sensations of labour are natural and the direct result of muscles working (and not an indication that something in her body is about to break), that she is safe and that she can do it, labour is usually manageable. A woman may need support to stay in the moment, to accept what is going on in her body, and help her muscles do their work by relaxing into the sensation of each contraction. When the body is producing an equal amount of oxytocin and endorphins, the experience is best described as intense muscle work, although it is bearable and manageable. There is no way around it: labour is a very intense experience, and a labouring woman can be compared to how someone might feel running a marathon or pushing themselves to the limit in another physical and mental way – but the sense of achievement and euphoria she feels when she finally gets to meet her baby is unlike anything else in life.

This is when a woman gets the opportunity to really get to know herself better and to find out what her body and mind are capable of. I can only describe this as an incredible gift that so many women are unaware of, and therefore overlook. The most helpful thing is to surrender or 'let go' to the sensation, to remain flexible and flowing, rather than rigid and stuck in wanting it to be a certain way.

How do women behave in labour?
Women behave in many different ways during labour. I love this quote by Phyllis Klaus: 'Labour is one of the most absorbing of human experiences,' as I think it really expresses what childbirth can be like. It is all-consuming, all-absorbing and a very intense experience – but also, in my view, one of the most insightful moments a woman can have. All the ups and downs of the different hormone surges, moments of intense muscle work (which translate as pain for many women), emotional outbursts and switches from one emotional state to another. A woman can be laughing and cracking jokes at one point in labour, and the next moment become anxious and childlike. At other times she might be angry and push her birth partners away, very soon after wanting them near her

and needing them to reassure her. She might swear, curse and appear angry and irritated, as well as have moments of self-doubt, crying and wanting to go home. These are the times when a woman is given the opportunity to learn more about herself and find the inner strength she might not know she possesses.

The day a woman gives birth to her baby is not just another day in her life, and it is therefore vital that she takes into account any events in her life that might have an impact on the birth. We all carry around memories, not only in our minds but also in our bodies, from all our life experiences, and often women in labour display a number of body memory-releasing behaviours. Below are some I have witnessed women doing during my work as a doula.

Emotions
Crying, sobbing, giggling, swearing, laughing, wanting her mum, whispering to the baby, talking to herself, calling for help, saying she's dying, saying she can't do it, wailing.

Movements
Shaking, clenching, grimacing, contorting her body, stiffness, quick walking, rocking from side to side, lifting alternative legs high in the air, standing with her forehead against a wall, swaying, standing on tiptoe, stretching her arms up above her head, lying completely still on her side.

Sounds
Sighing, groaning, moaning, grunting, growling, chanting, making vowel sounds, screaming, shouting, mooing.

What I believe to be absolutely crucial is that a woman giving birth feels safe to express all these different kinds of behaviours, as this helps her to release what might be in her body from a previous experience and helps her to birth her baby. If she feels she needs to remain in control, she will activate her neocortex (or intelligent brain; the area of the brain that she needs to shut down for physiological birth to unfold). This could lead to the whole process turning into suffering. If there is one thing I could prevent, it is seeing women suffering in childbirth – or at any other time, for that matter.

Why many women want a physiological birth

A spontaneous, straightforward physiological birth produces all the endogenous hormones designed to make the birth manageable for the woman, and also has a positive effect on the baby. Oxytocin and endorphins prepare the baby to breathe independently and to be able to regulate its body temperature after birth. As long as labour and birth continue undisturbed, they will also enable and trigger the spontaneous birth reflex. This birth reflex was named (by Dr Michel Odent) the *foetal ejection reflex*, and recently the word 'maternal' has been added to make it the *maternal foetal ejection reflex*. This makes it clear that the baby doesn't eject itself without the mother's help. It is the birthing woman who connects with this primal energy and allows the baby to be born. Dr Odent discovered that, at a certain time after the cervix is fully open, the birthing woman experiences her contractions differently: her body is opening up while a strong force is moving her baby downwards. This reflex has the same biological chain of events as vomiting, but in the opposite direction. It is a natural response very similar to a reverse sneeze, or the way our body moves food through the digestive system.

The maternal foetal ejection reflex is a natural reflex which will happen regardless of the wishes of the birthing woman, and is often described by women as an overwhelming, uncontrollable urge to push. After this reflex, labour will usually move along very quickly and the baby is soon born. This reflex is only activated during undisturbed and physiological childbirth – and, as it is there to be triggered, one could ponder on what impact it has on the mother and the baby if it is not utilised? I often wonder if we know how we might be altering the human race by interfering with a system we do not fully understand.

For the baby, the journey through the birth canal squeezes any liquid out of her lungs so that she can take her first breath as soon as she is born. Study after study has been carried out showing that, for both mother and baby, a physiological birth has many benefits. They all show that maternal and neonatal (mother and baby) mortality rates are lower after a physiological birth. Babies born physiologically and without any pain medication are statistically proven to be more alert and responsive (Romano, 2008).

Medications used during labour can have a variety of negative effects on the baby, including lowered heart rate, difficulty breathing, and lowered breastfeeding success after birth. Other studies have shown an increased likelihood of drug addiction in babies born after their mothers had pain medication during labour (Jacobson et al., 1990).

The benefits of physiological birth for the mother mean she will recover more quickly and easily, and that there will be no interference in the natural production of hormones, which means less risk that she will develop postnatal illness. Emerging research is suggesting that the use of synthetic oxytocin during childbirth may affect the endogenous oxytocin system, which could have an impact on the woman's stress levels, mood and behaviour (Bell et al., 2014). However, a physiological birth does not only have a positive impact in the immediate period after birth, but also has many long-term advantages. One of the knock-on effects from a medicated, high-tech birth include making breastfeeding harder – or even impossible – to establish, which will impact on how the woman feels about herself and could lead to a lack of self-esteem, which is difficult to measure. All the wonderful benefits of breastfeeding for both mother and baby might also be missed out, and this has a massive impact in the long term on the family and the generations to follow. These benefits are too many to list here, but a great resource can be downloaded by following this link. This document is based on research evidence with clear links to the actual data: www.infactcanada.ca/RisksofFormulaFeeding.pdf.

Most of us also have a great sense of wanting things to come 'full circle', or a need for there to be a completion of events in our lives. The birth process is designed to be a complete circle, enabling all the naturally occurring birth hormones to flow through the mother and baby, triggering the innate reflexes to ensure the optimal start for the new mother, her baby and the rest of the family. The focus of maternity care should be on enabling and facilitating physiological birth, not on lowering Caesarean birth rates. Women should be given good and solid research to enable them to choose the best place for them to feel safe to birth their baby. We should focus on what we want – not on what we *don't* want. I believe that if women were trusted and supported to make their own choices, with no value judgements on whether this is 'right' or 'wrong', and the only thing that mattered was how the women themselves felt about their choice, more women would have positive birth experiences.

The benefits of a medical birth

There will always be women and babies who will require the support and interventions of obstetric care when a pregnancy has complications and when a physiological birth is not possible, for whatever reason. There are rare, but real, emergencies that require swift action to save lives, and there are other common pregnancy-related illnesses which require intervention and treatment to ensure there is no permanent damage caused, such as pre-eclampsia, gestational diabetes, Strep B infections and obstetric cholestasis.

A woman should never be forced into having a physiological birth or a medicalised birth. After learning about all the benefits and risks associated with both options, she should be free to make an informed choice. However, for an informed choice to be made, the information needs to be provided in an objective way and based on the best available research – and not on the opinions of one expert.

Some women who have suffered previous traumas, such as survivors of sexual abuse or sufferers of tocophobia (a fear of childbirth), might only be able to give birth to their baby with the support and aid of pain management and obstetric procedures. However, there is no guaranteed way of giving birth that does not come without the possibility of trauma, mostly depending on how the woman is treated and is feeling during the process. Woman can be traumatised during a medical birth as well as during physiological childbirth. The focus must always be on fully listening to and emotionally connecting with what the woman is saying, and her reasons for wanting her birth to be a certain way. Care providers need to be respectful of all choices!

The main benefit of a medical birth is that it results in a healthy mother and baby – and, hopefully, the woman felt part of her birth experience and was able to participate in decision-making, or at least be included in discussions around her care. A medical birth also often prevents women from suffering, and also from trauma. In a true emergency, a medical birth saves lives.

However, we must remain cautious, and consider whether all medical births really needed to go down this route. I believe that inductions for overdue babies (postdates), Caesarean births for breech babies and multiple pregnancies, restrictions for women because they are over a certain age, and other guidelines that do not take into account the individual woman and her circumstances should be changed to include a more holistic and human-centred approach. Health care professionals must stop playing the 'dead baby' card and instead present information in an objective way, as well as giving the risks associated with many medical procedures. Women should be given the chance to make the right decision for them and their babies, even if her wishes go against what the clinical guidelines are saying.

Considerations for the birth partner
I believe one of the biggest challenges for a birth partner is to be able to accept physiological childbirth as a natural process. The birth-giver will be going through the mental and physical challenges that are involved in a physiological birth. These are all part of the process and no solutions can usually be offered. If I can pass on any message to a potential birth partner, it is this: it cannot be fixed! It might seem logical to think that if the pain is taken away, it will make birth a better experience for the woman, but very often this 'fix' is to make it a better experience for the birth partner, who might be finding it difficult to watch and support the woman he loves in labour. A birth partner will see their loved one acting and behaving in a way that they have probably never seen before, and this can feel very scary, and even a bit disturbing. It is normal to see the woman completely naked – not only in the sense of having no clothes or make-up on, but seeing her core being as a primal mammal. She will seem to have lost her mind at times; she might express herself very primally with one-word communication; she might sound as though she is having

sex, moaning and sighing; and she may swear and curse and push her birth partner away. I often hear birth partners believing that the woman is 'on another planet' and detached from what is happening in the room, which is what it might look like. However, a woman in labour is very sensitive to her environment and will subconsciously hear and notice everything that is going on.

It is really important not to feel sorry for the woman in labour, as she needs to have solid support and the belief and faith of her birth partner that she can do it. When things get tough and she is expressing how hard it is for her, her feelings need to be acknowledged, not dismissed. It is not helpful to tell a woman in labour who is saying that she can't do it that thousands of women have given birth before her, so of course she can do it. It's better if a birth partner can acknowledge that things are really tough for her right now and reassure her that she is doing an amazing job and everyone believes in her. Women don't always require a fix for their problems; often, they simply want to be heard and have their feelings acknowledged. Often this enables and energises a woman to carry on and break through this difficult part of labour and reach a new level of strength.

Sometimes in labour, women enjoy being touched and massaged, but this can change very quickly. What might have felt good five minutes ago may all of a sudden be painful or irritating. In labour, women are usually only able to express that they want the massage to stop by putting their hand out, pushing their birth partner's hand away, or shouting 'Stop'. This can make the birth partner feel rejected or even make them feel bad that they don't know what to do to help their loved one. It's helpful to remember that a woman in labour is behaving in a primal way, so all the social niceties are gone. This should be seen as a good sign that she is deep in her primal brain, and that labour is probably going very well. Consider the same thing when women get angry and annoyed with their birth partner. It is important to bring along an 'emotional waste bin' where the birth partner can dump any feelings of being under attack when the way the birthing woman is behaving is upsetting, even though this is absolutely normal during childbirth. Staying close to the woman will be comforting, and it is always worth remembering that saying nothing is better than saying the wrong thing.

A woman in labour needs to be given unconditional love and support from her birth partners during the all-consuming experience of childbirth.

As a doula, I have witnessed a variety of births, many of which have been physiological births. When a woman is given the protective environment she needs, and the reassurance and love she requires, she often manages labour and birth very well. I see women glowing with oxytocin, deeply connected to their breathing and following their body's guidance, telling them what position to be in. I'm always in awe at the amazing power that women have within themselves, and the way they grow and move to a higher level during labour and birth.

MAKE IT REAL

You may like to think about, or discuss with your birth partner, the following.

How you could encourage oxytocin during labour: What makes you feel good? Perhaps it is a certain smell or music? Could you bring your own blanket with you to hospital to make it feel more like home? What about lighting – how could you light your chosen birth environment? (Birth centres and hospitals will allow you to bring electric candles, for example.) If massage makes you feel relaxed, perhaps your birth partner could learn some simple massage techniques. Write a list of things that will encourage oxytocin and keep adrenaline at bay.

If you have a birth partner, do they understand what is normal behaviour in labour and birth?

You might also be interested in taking a pregnancy yoga, hypnobirthing or meditation class to help you feel connected to your body and more able to listen to it. These classes encourage you to relax and let go during labour, embracing the physiological process as natural and normal.

Secret #3
You don't need to study for childbirth - it's all within you.

ᘓᘔᘓ

Chapter 3: Influencers on Childbirth

I often wonder whether pregnant women who watch TV programmes or read books about childbirth are aware of the risks they might be taking by using an academic approach to birth. Is it possible to lose intuition and gut feeling by relying too much on information and knowledge? Does it create an imbalance in the mind and a disconnection from the body? Women are so used to preparing for big events in their lives, such as exams, weddings and job interviews, that they have started to rely more on 'facts and figures' than intuitive knowledge. Women are also choosing to have children later in life, when they have established a good career and a lifestyle and daily pattern with which they are comfortable and used to leading. They see having a baby as the next thing in their life plan, and very often continue working until a couple of weeks before their baby is due.

Preparing for the birth of a child requires a woman to listen to her body and to start connecting with the baby as soon as she is aware that she is pregnant. We know from research that a baby is very aware in the womb, and from around twenty weeks' gestation can hear everything that goes on around them. There are many benefits to be gained from singing, talking and connecting to the baby during pregnancy – for both the mother and the baby. It's often difficult for women to be 'present' in their body and really feel and notice what is going on. Many women don't notice that their baby is moving throughout the day, and perhaps having hiccups on a regular basis. Others don't recollect feeling the practice tightenings, called Braxton Hicks, which are there to prepare the uterus for labour. I often see a disconnection between the mother-to-be and her unborn baby, as if the baby is not real until it has been born. This is particularly true when working with couples who have had IVF (in vitro fertilisation) treatment. I guess it must be a natural way of protecting themselves from disappointment, as many IVF treatments end in failure or miscarriage, so many couples undergoing IVF must feel fearful of falling in love with their unborn child until they know it is going to survive. I have huge admiration and compassion for these couples.

The aim for anyone who wants to educate and support pregnant women before, during and after birth is to ask themselves if what they are teaching is best for the women, or if what they are teaching is simply to reinforce or justify their own opinions or expertise.

Various products and services that have been attached to the notion of emotional security through advertising and promotion are making huge financial profits based on women's need to feel in control. I would put some hypnobirthing companies and antenatal preparation services in this category, as well as personal baby heart rate monitors and a number of other baby products. The reliance on external resources and input from experts could actually be undermining women's belief that childbirth is normal and physiological. It's forcing the woman to look outside her body and its abilities, and placing greater emphasis on the importance of external paraphernalia to give birth, when the focus should be on herself.

What if a woman has experienced abuse?
If a woman has experienced any kind of abuse, physical, mental or sexual, this will most likely have an impact on the birth process. Many of the processes and sensations women feel during childbirth – and procedures by medical professionals – can feel similar to what they experienced during the abuse. If a woman is committed to giving birth physiologically, she needs to know that it can involve hard work, and

requires a whole lot of determination, the right support people around her, and an openness to accepting what unfolds in the process. The physical memory of the abuse in the woman's body will usually not just go away, and often it can't be overcome by positive thinking alone. It has to be dealt with by some type of healing or therapy. This requires a lot of bravery and it can be a challenging journey for the woman.

The women I have supported who were survivors of sexual abuse all had good birth experiences, even though they found it tough at times, as they had spent time working with a therapist to get some of their issues resolved before the birth. They were able to become aware of their 'triggers' and we worked on ways to minimise these during labour and birth. These women were able to trust in their bodies again and relax into the sensations that labour brings. The feeling of being out of control, of people in authority asking to do things to them, about being naked and feeling something inside them that is painful did not make them relive their abuse, or traumatise them; instead, the birth was a healing experience for them. They pushed their pain out with their baby.

Everyone will relate to and feel pain differently. Some women will even experience the baby moving around in labour as pain, probably because they are in a state of fear, registering everything that is happening in their body as a sign of something being wrong. I have seen survivors of abuse be hypersensitive to every bodily sensation, thus making it very difficult for them to switch off and trust what is happening in their body and to see it as being a good thing. I can imagine it is difficult to trust your body when it has let you down before, and also to be comfortable with the sensations that are felt in the areas of the body that have been 'shut down' as a survival mechanism to handle the previous trauma.

I don't think physiological childbirth is necessarily the right thing for all women, as I don't want to see any women suffer in childbirth. Sometimes it might be better to look at what is possible in terms of the journey of self-discovery and healing. For some women, it might just not be the right time, or they might not have enough time to achieve enough self-awareness to go through the necessary process of transformation before facing childbirth. Trying to relax into a physiological birth when the body's memory is expecting pain and your whole being is anticipating the next sensations by fighting back (in the form of adrenaline production) makes labour more painful and more drawn-out. Women must understand that what has happened to them in the past will not stay in the past during childbirth and motherhood. Instead, this can be viewed as an opportunity to heal from the past and come out the other side stronger and whole. However, the woman has to decide for herself if she is willing to start that journey. It usually isn't that simple, as recognising that there is an issue and then taking the necessary steps towards healing can be extremely frightening. It is key that she finds a therapist or healer who specialises in trauma that she can fully trust.

Hypnobirthing

There are a number of different companies that produce hypnobirthing CDs to listen to during pregnancy. Their purpose is to learn to manage childbirth with the help of hypnotherapy and exercises. I think hypnobirthing is a great tool for couples to add to their 'toolbox' when preparing for the birth of their baby; however, it can also be a bit misleading if it is sold as *the* way to give birth without feeling any pain. I'm also very aware that if a couple have done hypnobirthing and the woman is still experiencing pain or is unable to use the exercises in labour, it is easy to place the blame on her – 'she's probably not doing it right!'

The other thing to consider with hypnobirthing is that some of the pre-written relaxation scripts might not be suitable for the women who are listening to them. Imagine a woman listening to a script that describes a beautiful, sandy beach, with the sound of waves lapping against the shore, the smell of the sea air and the warm sun on her skin. If this woman happens to have had a very unpleasant experience on a beach, perhaps being attacked or raped, she will probably not feel very relaxed and might even end up having a panic attack. Any script that is not created and written by the couple themselves could be a potential trigger for any recent memories or old childhood memories that have been repressed.

Women who are survivors of childhood sexual abuse often have no memory of it: a normal way for the body to handle trauma is to hide it away in the back of our minds. To be brought back into a place or location where the abuse took place, which others assume is a safe place, could be a disaster for the woman, her partner and the hypnobirthing teacher. It is therefore probably best if the couple create their own scripts and safe places for use during the birth process.

I also believe that it is better to make sure that women expect to feel some intense sensations during labour and childbirth, and to realise that they may be experienced as pain. Women will interpret these sensations in their own way; some will say that it was excruciating, while others will say that the sensations were enjoyable, or even orgasmic. It is unfair to tell women that if they practise hypnobirthing, they will feel no pain, as this might not be true for all women.

Active birth

Women are often told that when they are in labour, they should remain active and not lie down, as keeping active means that gravity will aid the birth process. Women have been taught to squat during labour, and remain upright. By telling women that one way of birthing is better than another, we stop them from listening to their own bodies and doing what is best for them as an individual. As all women give birth differently, surely all women need to be in a position that works for them and to do what they need to do in labour? What works for one woman may not work for another, so there is no 'one size fits all' approach.

When I listen to birth stories, I often hear about women who have woken up early in the morning a few days past their estimated due date, usually around 2 a.m., due to some tightenings of their womb. They have learnt in their antenatal classes that they need to be active in labour so they immediately get out of bed and start walking around. They keep walking until 7 a.m., when the tightenings fade away and stop, by which time they are feeling tired and despondent. Often the woman starts thinking that there is something wrong with her body and her baby will never come out. The following night labour starts again and this time it's the real thing. She will be tired due to lack of sleep from the previous night, and she will not be in the best state of mind to begin her journey to meet her baby. It would have been better for her to stay in bed until she felt she needed to get up, rather than following a prescriptive, learnt pattern.

If we look at physiological birth, we understand that we need to increase the release of hormones such as oxytocin and endorphins during labour. We also know that we should keep adrenaline at bay as, overall, this is not a good hormone during childbirth, especially during dilation of the cervix. A woman who wants to lie down, usually on her side, is most likely producing less adrenaline than a woman who is making herself walk around because she has been taught that this is best for giving birth. I don't disagree that gravity can be very helpful, but this is when things are not progressing as expected during a physiological birth. I feel we should only offer suggestions to women at a time when they might feel unsure of what position to be in. If labour is slowing down and there are real reasons why the baby has to be born sooner rather than later, using gravity can be very helpful. This is when making suggestions and supporting the labouring woman to try something new can be a good idea.

I have supported women who have not moved at all during labour, apart from to go to the bathroom. They have lain on their side, resting in between and breathing through the contractions, totally relaxed. When the urge to push came, they just lifted their leg and had a baby. As simple as that! If a woman is in labour, she is in labour. It can't be speeded up, forced or controlled, and a woman will usually intuitively know what she needs to do to manage her baby's birth. She will choose a position that is good for her; she will birth in the time she needs to adjust mentally to becoming a mother; and she will birth her baby in her own unique way. All that is normally required is strong, solid support from trusted birth professionals who are willing to give her the time she needs to birth her baby.

If women are constantly bombarded by advice and ordered around in labour, it is more likely to cause confusion and a conflict within, especially if the woman can't do what she feels like doing. This might lead to elevated levels of adrenaline, which would be counterproductive during a physiological birth. Feeling annoyed or irritated in labour is not supporting or encouraging the hormones needed, and it also keeps the woman in her thinking brain.

Communication

Communication is a two-way system in which someone talks and the other party listens. Everyone hears what is being said differently, depending on their culture, life experience and current state of mind. I can be talking to a group of twenty people, and they will all interpret and process the information I'm sharing with them in their own unique way. This means they will also make up their own story and create a memory of what I said, based on any knowledge they already have, and experiences that are similar to what I'm talking to them about.

When we experience something that evokes an emotional response, we are trying to make sense of the situation and will do this by making up a 'story' based on what we already know. This means that a lot of the birth stories women are told by other women don't make sense and are often factually incorrect. What we hear is how this woman experienced the birth of her baby and, after telling it many times, having solutions and fixes added by those around her, she has created a story which makes sense to her and fills in all the gaps. I'm not suggesting she is lying or making things up; we still must listen to her story and acknowledge her feelings. What I am saying is that what we're hearing is how *she* experienced her birth and how *she* has since made sense of it. It is not necessarily exactly what happened; instead, it is her interpretation of it.

When we communicate with women before, during and after childbirth, we need to be very sensitive with the words we use, the way we put our information across, and the tone of voice in which we communicate. Women are extremely sensitive to anything that might sound judgemental or harsh, or come across as criticism.

The words we use when communicating, especially during pregnancy and birth, have a huge impact on women, the way they feel about their bodies and their ability to give birth. Being mindful of the way we communicate is such a simple thing, and can have such a huge impact.

My children used to sing a song at assembly when they were at primary school, and some of the words went: 'Your tongue's a tiny part of your body, but such enormous harm can be done by it. Every time you open your mouth, you've got to think before you speak.' I think the text is wonderful, and simply explains how careful we should be with the words we use.

In the antenatal period

When women are told that they have developed a pregnancy-related problem, the information they are given is often confusing for them, and may be delivered in a manner that can leave them stressed and upset. The perceived risk of something going wrong is often not very clearly expressed, and data and statistics are often misunderstood by the pregnant woman. Instead of offering real numbers to compare, statistics are often communicated as 'double the chance' or 'increased risks'. If something doubles from something that was small in the first place, there isn't much of an increased risk. Women need to have clear and simple information so that they understand the situation rather than the emotional blackmail that sometimes takes place. If the risk factor is 5 in 1,000, it might be easier for a woman to understand if it is also presented as a 0.5% risk or, even better, a 99.5% chance of it *not* happening. To make a sweeping statement that there is an increased risk of having a baby that is unwell or stillborn naturally frightens the woman and she will be unable to think rationally about how to proceed.

Most of the time, there is also no mention of the risks associated with medical interventions, such as the increased risks in a Caesarean birth after a medically induced induction of labour (Vardo et al., 2011). Or that routine clinical guidelines, such as continuous foetal monitoring during labour for women with low-risk pregnancies, increase the chances of a Caesarean birth by 20% – with no known evidence that there are any benefits for doing this (Devane et al., 2017).

Here's an example. A client of mine went to see her midwife, who measured her pregnant belly and told her she was measuring big for her dates at thirty-six weeks. She was sent to the hospital for a weight scan of the baby and a glucose test. Her glucose levels were found to be borderline high, so she was referred to a consultant. The consultant told her that *if* she had gestational diabetes, her chances of a traumatic birth would increase and the baby could become unwell; then, in the next sentence, he said that a baby who measured large on a scan was not an indication that something had to be done about it. He then told her he'd see her in two weeks and to go home and not worry about it! I think this is possibly the worst thing anyone can say in such a situation – as it indicates that there *is* something to worry about.

My client *did* worry that the baby would get even bigger over the next couple of weeks and about what would happen if that was the case. She was never officially diagnosed with gestational diabetes and, during labour, no one even mentioned her glucose levels, but her meeting with the consultant had a huge impact on her mentally. She stopped eating (to prevent the baby from getting any bigger, as she was worried about making the baby huge). When labour started, her body was already in ketosis (that is, she had no energy stores for labour and needed an intravenous drip of fluids). Her birth took a completely different route than she had hoped for, and I'm sure that her meeting with the consultant hugely impacted on her birth.

If he had been more mindful of the way he was communicating with the pregnant woman sitting in front of him, things could have been very different. When medical staff are simply following a set of written guidelines without engaging with their patient on an emotional level, much damage can be done. Of course, they need to convey what they need to, but should always remember what the potential impact could be on their 'patient'. Women listen with their hearts when they are pregnant, so only need to hear what is going to be helpful to them and relevant at the time. Information should, of course, not be kept from a pregnant woman, but the way it is presented and communicated should be a priority.

In labour
Words can mean so many different things to different people, and having the sensitivity to consider how we say things could prevent someone from suffering unnecessarily or reliving a trauma. We all have words that

'trigger' reactions in us in one way or another, and different words can be triggers to different people.

Penny Simkin and Phyllis Klaus, in their book *When Survivors Give Birth*, explain that especially during times of stress, the words and actions of a caregiver can elicit unexpected behaviours in childhood abuse survivors.

They list the following phrases, usually said to be helpful but which could potentially be the same words that are used by an abuser:

> 'Open your legs'
> 'Relax your bottom'
> 'This will hurt only a little'
> 'Relax, and it won't hurt so much'
> (Simkin and Klaus, 2004)

If any words or phrases are being said to you in labour that make you feel uncomfortable, it is important that you tell your caregivers immediately. There should be no need to add lengthy explanations for why certain words should not be used: a simple, 'Don't say that, I don't like it' should be enough. It might even be a better idea to put these phrases/words in your birth preferences document beforehand, so that they're in writing and your birth partner can remind the other caregivers of them.

Other words can also act as triggers, or are better not to be used, and these are listed below.

Words that disempower and criticise the woman's body:

- Caesarean section – we talk about people with mental illness being 'sectioned'
- delivery/delivered – as many people have said before, pizzas are delivered, babies are birthed!
- pain relief – it sounds as though the pain is a bad thing and needs to be taken away
- contractions – something is being pulled together; sounds painful

- failure to progress – this implies it is the woman's fault that she is not progressing in labour
- lack of maternal effort – sounds as if the woman can't be bothered to birth her baby
- incompetent cervix – the woman's body is failing
- lazy uterus – the woman's body is failing.

Words to use instead:
- Caesarean birth – refers to a baby being born, rather than a woman 'sectioned'; sounds more active
- Birth/birthed – the woman always births her baby; no one delivers it
- Pain management – sounds more positive, as if the pain can be managed
- Surges/rushes – talks about the hormones surging, causing the uterus to work.

A woman's body very rarely 'fails' to give birth to her baby, but often she does not get the right support and is not giving birth in an environment in which she feels safe. Any phrases referring to the woman's body failing are better labelled as an 'unsupportive environment'.

Phrases and words randomly used when supporting women in labour and birth could bring back bad memories, or memories she has hidden away in the back of her mind. We are as we are for a reason and, at times, birth professionals and birth partners might be the target for a labouring woman's unexpressed feelings. However, the birthing woman needs empathy and compassion, not harsh words or punishment for not complying.

In the postnatal period
As a doula course facilitator, I have read over a thousand birth stories. As a doula, I have seen first-hand what well-meaning hospital staff, partners and family members say to women who have just had a baby.

A story I have heard many times is about a new mum in hospital who puts her baby on her bed without making sure she can't roll off, and is told off by a member of staff for not keeping her baby safe. Also, women are often given overwhelming and confusing information about breastfeeding. For many women, being told off when they have just started out as a mother can have a long-lasting effect on how they feel about themselves as a competent mother. It's a confusing time and, as a new mother finds her feet and her own ways of being a mum, she needs to be talked to with kindness and gentleness.

There are guidelines and recommendation for keeping a baby safe, but there is no reason why these can't be communicated in a caring manner. No new mother should be told off for doing the best she can with the information that she has at the time. Time and time again, women tell me how they can remember when someone said something mean to them during birth or in the postnatal period. It is difficult for new mums not to take to heart things that have been said to them when their bodies are aching, their lives have been turned upside down, and they are desperate for some nurturing and kindness.

If women expect to encounter people who are not going to say helpful things in the postnatal period, they can choose to ignore what is said to them. If women realised that *they* are the experts on how to look after their baby, they can choose what information they take on board and what to ignore, and trust their instincts.

Making a choice

I often hear women say that they are 'not allowed' to choose certain things in their pregnancy: for example, they 'have to' be induced or they 'weren't allowed' to give birth at home. It is often a misinterpretation of what they have heard that makes them come to this conclusion. Everyone is free to make their own choices about their upcoming birth and postnatal period; however, women often believe that someone else knows better than them, and women might also feel it is a huge responsibility to live with the choices they make. What if they make the wrong decision and something goes wrong with the birth? I prefer to talk about *choices* rather than *decisions*, and what is so wonderful about this way of talking is that a woman can choose one thing at one moment, based on the information she has at the time and on how she is feeling. Things might change, and then the woman can make a different choice. Nothing needs to be final, and at no point does she have to make a decision. Women need to connect with their hearts and really feel what is right for them and their babies. What often is lacking is someone who can support them in their decision-making and act as a sounding board for their intuitive feelings and knowledge.

It's easy to think – and believe – that we are not choosing to react angrily if someone has insulted us, or not choosing to react positively when someone has paid us a compliment. We tend to think that someone else has made us react in the ways we react, and that we have not made a conscious choice. In fact, we all respond to most situations automatically, like Pavlov's dog, who salivates when the bell is rung as he has associated the sound with the arrival of food. Women have been so conditioned by what they have seen in the media and what they have heard friends and family tell them about childbirth that their responses and choices are often clouded by incorrect information. We are all always free to choose how to react to what is said to us and what we are experiencing.

It is important for women to take a step back and really look at the choices they are making. By doing that, they will become aware of whether they are simply reacting automatically or choosing for themselves. Many women have stopped listening to their intuition, that primal gut feeling, and are often worried about getting things wrong or making a rod for their own backs. Many would sooner trust the experts than make a decision for themselves and their baby.

Making choices by listening to what your body is telling you is not complicated. Usually when you make a decision you will have a 'gut feeling' about the right thing to do, and when you have chosen that option, you will feel (around your heart or solar plexus) comfort and a good sensation. If you feel discomfort or unease, then perhaps you have made the wrong choice. Studies have been carried out that look at the way our 'gut' talks directly to our brain, and scientists believe our 'gut instinct' is an old warning system which has evolved to help the human race survive. Our 'gut instinct' is a physiological response and should not be ignored. Whatever the message your body is sending back to you, it is important to pay attention to it. The slightest feeling of discomfort could indicate that the choice you are about to make is the wrong one. Women need to start believing in their innate knowledge and intuitive nature so that they can make choices confidently.

Women are often given information during pregnancy that is not always based on evidence or clinical trials and because women have become so unsure and mistrusting of their own bodies, they believe that the expert knows more than they do. A recent study found that 'fewer than 20% of recommendations by the RCOG (Royal College of Obstetricians and Gynaecologists) were based on high-quality evidence, with a large proportion based on "recommended best practice" and expert opinion' (Prusova, 2014). Due to this growing culture of 'expert opinion', many women have stopped listening to and trusting their bodies, and this intrinsic feedback system is often overridden. Instead they will go with what the expert is telling them.

Women should be aware that they can trust their heart and their body's response, as it is rare for this to be wrong. Doctors recognise this intuitive connection the woman has with her baby, and will often tell women that if they feel that something is wrong with them or their baby, they should contact their midwife. It's not something that can be measured scientifically, but that doesn't mean it is not real. Many women will 'just know' that there is something wrong. I wish that the same trust could be placed in women when they make decisions about how they want to birth their baby.

The challenge of saying 'no'
From a very early age, girls are taught to be 'good' and are encouraged and rewarded for following the instructions of someone in authority. It is so ingrained in our society that most of us don't even know it is happening. Little girls are meant to be sweet and good, while little boys are allowed to be boisterous and challenging. When girls behave like boys they are often labelled as 'bossy' or described as a 'tomboy'. Because most women have grown up aiming to be good girls, it is often very difficult to

challenge what someone in authority is telling them to do, especially when they are being told about the perceived safety and health of their baby.

Women have the responsibility of carrying a baby in their womb, and because of the negative language around women's bodies generally, it can feel very scary for women to take responsibility for the way they birth their baby. At times it can seem as though there are too many 'what ifs'. When women are presented with information that is given in a confusing way, it's no surprise that women say they felt they had no choice about what course of action to take. It can also make giving birth seem a lot riskier than it really is. Generally speaking, birth is 99% safe if the woman has had a trouble-free pregnancy – and this is a fact (Birthplace in England Collaborative Group, 2011). 'White coat syndrome' and the way we act and behave around someone in authority can transform even the most assertive woman into a compliant and trusting 'patient'. The phrase, 'trust me, I'm a doctor' is fresh in women's minds, and they think, 'Why would a doctor not do what is best for me and my baby?'

A very simple decision-making tool when you're faced with making a choice about a test or intervention is the BRAIN model. BRAIN stands for Benefits, Risks, Alternatives, Intuition – and it also considers what will happen if you do Nothing.

For example, if you are being offered an induction of labour as you have gone past your estimated due date, you can ask yourself what the Benefits of this would be. Find out if there are any Risks associated with an induction of labour and whether there are any Alternatives. Spend a moment tuning into what your Intuition, or gut feeling, is about the induction. You can also ask your care providers what would happen if you choose to do Nothing.

I would like to see women across the globe starting to accept that they know best and that they have full autonomy over their bodies. This would lead to women starting to act on what their instincts are telling them, and do what feels right, rather than blindly trust what an expert might be telling them.

It is completely fine to ask for time alone to discuss and consider any medical intervention with a birth partner as well as asking midwives and doctors to explain in more detail any potential risks of a suggested procedures – and how these could affect your labour and the birth of your baby. It is also OK to ask if the situation is a medical emergency or whether it's feasible to wait and see how things progress. You are absolutely within your rights to ask for clarification, facts and figures before you make a choice.

I believe women will only be able to stand up for themselves when they realise just how powerful they are and that their bodies are amazing. When statistics and risk factors are presented in a clear and objective way and care providers offer the treatment or intervention as a real option which the woman can feel free and comfortable to decline. When women also can see that to give birth to a baby is an experience that can be transformational and something to be excited about doing. That is when women will be able to take responsibility for their own births and birth *their* way.

MAKE IT REAL

You may like to think about, or discuss with your birth partner, the following.

Whether you feel that extra birth preparation classes, such as hypnobirthing or active birth classes, are right for you.

How language can affect birth, and if there is any language you would like your midwives and other care providers to avoid during your labour. Some women add to their birth preferences that they would prefer their midwife to avoid certain words ('pain' or 'contraction', for example) and choose instead 'comfort' or 'surge'.

What tools and information will you use if you need to make potentially difficult choices during labour? How comfortable does your birth partner feel about advocating for you?

If you are a survivor of abuse, now is the time to make contact with a therapist (your GP may be able to refer you) for support before you go into labour. You may also want to consider whether you would like to prepare for a physiological birth, or plan for an elective Caesarean birth.

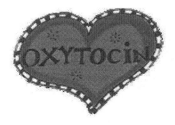

Secret #4

Childbirth changes a woman's view of herself.

CR80

Chapter 4: The Impact of Birthing on a Woman

Giving birth, which is a natural process, has (since it moved from the home into hospital) become very medicalised. It's spoken about as dangerous, painful and not to be attempted without expert advice. The language used by obstetricians about pregnancy and birth is very different from the language that women speak. When doctors talk about a pregnancy being 'high risk', a labour being 'prolonged', a woman having an 'inadequate pelvis' or an 'incompetent cervix', they present a view of the world – and the place of women in it – that imposes a certain set of values and which assumes that they, as scientists, can step back and make judgements separate from the objects and systems they study (Kitzinger, 1999). Women, therefore, often believe that it's better and safer to give birth in a hospital, where they will be protected from these perceived dangers and pains of childbirth and be assisted with their 'malfunctioning' bodies.

Medical tests and diagnoses made by experts are assumed to be more accurate and more important than the emotional wellbeing of the woman. A woman who is very assertive when operating in her own world often becomes disempowered in the hospital environment where power is usually associated with the medical staff and their expertise. The use of pain management might provide a woman with the sense that she is in control – but it could also be used to the advantage of the hospital, to make the woman quiet and compliant. Tests and expert involvement are rarely questioned, and are often just taken for granted. The consequence of this is that the woman's perceived lack of agency has an emotional cost, and can create a sense of failure of being a woman and a mother.

I believe that a woman's experience when she gives birth to her children has a direct impact on the rest of her life. All too often, I notice how unaware not only women are about this, but the majority of the population. A study carried out by Birthrights through Mumsnet showed that 63% of women agreed that their births had an impact on how they felt about themselves, and a negative birth experience gets motherhood off to a bad start (Birthrights, 2013). If you have a bad birth experience, you have a higher risk of suffering postnatal illness, such as post-traumatic stress disorder (PTSD) and depression. It could also impact on the success a woman has with breastfeeding which, over the long term, has been shown to affect both a baby's and a mother's health.

Giving birth is so interwoven with the identity of being a woman that it's not surprising that it can alter a woman's self-image. When people talk about birth as being a 'natural' event and when women feel that they did not have the birth they hoped for, they might also feel that they are different to – and worse than – women who gave birth the way nature intended. This may lead to them feeling 'unnatural'. As giving birth to a baby is a huge part of being a woman, they start doubting everything about themselves – their very 'woman-ness'. Births with a lot of interventions or births ending in a Caesarean often impact negatively on breastfeeding success, so not only does the woman feel like she has failed at giving birth, being unable to breastfeed is another thing that cements her belief that her body is not working properly: again, she has 'failed' at being a 'natural' woman and mother.

During pregnancy, women have to wait patiently for a whole nine months before they get to meet their baby – and sometimes even longer. I feel that Mother Nature is trying to teach them how to get used to the unpredictability of not knowing exactly when the baby is going to arrive.

When the baby finally arrives, each day with your newborn will be different, and if a woman can wake up each day and accept that it is pointless to struggle against what is happening, that having a baby means every day is as unpredictable as the estimated date of birth, she will be able to enjoy those first few precious weeks a whole lot more.

This can be extremely difficult for women who like to feel in control and plan their lives: women who make lists and always want to be one step ahead, knowing every possible outcome so that they can plan for every eventuality, often feel frustrated when they can't do this when they are planning for their birth. These women often say initially that they don't want to do something – for example, have their labour induced – but then when the time comes still choose this option, defending their decision with 'the doctor told me to'. Even if they are presented with evidence-based research that shows the opposite, they are often not open to considering this information. They feel in control and safe in the knowledge that they are basing their choice on what an 'expert' has said, ultimately not taking responsibility themselves. It is usually not until after the birth that they understand how their choice has impacted on their birth and they can see the full picture. If they feel that they were misled or not given adequate information, it can be hugely disappointing. Often this may lead to feelings of inadequacy and even postnatal illness.

I see that the struggle or conflict this can evoke comes from being unable to accept what the present moment holds – and the sooner a woman sees that she can do nothing about this, and surrenders to this new way of being, she can enjoy her pregnancy. I have worked with women who wanted to find out everything they could about things that could go wrong so that they could 'watch out' for these things and fix them before they occur. I am not against antenatal testing, but I think it is important to consider why you are taking the test and what decisions you might make based on the results. For example, if you are having tests for Down's syndrome, what would you do if the results of the test indicated that there was a very high chance of your child being born with this condition? Would you terminate the pregnancy or welcome your baby, no matter what? If your choice would be the latter, then why have the test?

Private 3D and 4D scans are becoming increasingly popular with pregnant couples, but a concern of mine is that no one actually knows for sure whether these scans are harmless. A statement was made by Public Health England on the use of ultrasound scans without any diagnostic purpose, simply to provide souvenir images or recordings of the unborn as keepsakes. They wrote:

> While there is no clear evidence that such exposures are harmful to the foetus, parents-to-be must decide for themselves whether they wish to have souvenir scans. The desire for the keepsake must be balanced against the possibility of unconfirmed risks to the unborn ... the HPA (the Health Protection Agency) is aware that research into the safety of ultrasound continues to be carried out both in the UK and abroad. In the light of the uncertainties surrounding the possibility of neurological effects from prenatal exposure, the HPA endorses the need for such research, particularly with regard to in utero exposures. (Public Health England, 2012)

During pregnancy, women are offered at least two ultrasound scans and they are usually carried out at eight to fourteen weeks and between eighteen and twenty weeks. The first scan is known as a dating scan, when the sonographer estimates the due date of the baby based on the baby's measurements. The second scan is called the anomaly scan and this scan checks for structural abnormalities (anomalies) in the baby.

I had a client who had a private scan at thirty-four weeks. During the scan, the sonographer noticed an anomaly with the baby's brain. This had not been picked up before and, after more than one 'second opinion', the doctors decided it had been a mistake and that the baby was healthy. However, the weeks that followed this scan were filled with worry and sadness, with the parents-to-be wondering whether the baby they had wanted so much was going to be born with brain damage. This impacted on the birth, as my client held back from letting her baby out, just in case the baby wasn't perfect! Luckily, when she eventually had her baby, it was a healthy and beautiful little girl. My client pondered, in hindsight, whether she should have paid for that extra scan: if she hadn't, she would have been none the wiser and she could have enjoyed her last weeks of pregnancy more. Who knows how different her birth might have been had she not gone into it full of worry and stress?

I really believe that pregnancy is designed to force people's patterns of behaviour to change, as life with a newborn requires a woman to be patient and to take each day as it comes.

It is the same when preparing for the birth. It will be what it will be, and in my view the only preparation that people need to do is to fully understand the physiology of birth. If giving birth in a hospital, understand how the system works, what options are available, know that you have the right to decline any treatment offered, and fully understand the impact of any pain medication and intervention, not only in the short term but also the long-term effects. I won't go on to list them all here, but a good article can be found on the AIMS website: www.aims.org.uk/effectDrugsOnBabies.htm. After that, you need to make sure that the environment you choose to give birth in is well protected and that you have the right people around you.

I've seen women in labour who are struggling to come to terms with the fact that the kind of person they thought they were and what they hoped they would be like in labour is not true for them at all. They may find it impossible to switch off their thinking brain; they may be unable to try any of the comfort measures (such as breathing techniques, visualisations and hypnobirthing scripts) they thought they'd like; they no longer want to take responsibility for their own birth – instead, they want someone to rescue them and tell them what to do.

In my view, there are few life experiences in which a woman gets to truly see who she is, and I think there are two ways to deal with a birth experience that did not turn out the way a woman had hoped for. The first option is to simply accept what has happened; accept that this is who she is. There's absolutely nothing wrong with realising that a physiological birth hasn't worked for her this time. The second option is to reflect and learn from the experience, and see where she would like to make some changes, where she could have chosen differently. This might seem an easy thing to do: however, I suspect that many women instead choose another option, which is to find someone to blame – usually themselves – for what happened to them. It is not surprising that they do, as everything around childbirth can be 'blamed' on the woman, as I mentioned earlier. The birth process cannot be taken out of the context of the woman's life; it impacts her on a deep level, consciously or unconsciously.

I believe women need to be more honest with themselves and with their care providers about what kind of a birth they think they would like – but also what kind of birth their body and mind can manage. There is a saying, 'we birth like we live', and I couldn't agree more. However, I would also like to add that everyone has the option to change how they live, and they can choose differently if they have the commitment and will to do so. For some women, to avoid suffering, it is best to give birth with some form of medical intervention such as pain management or continuous monitoring, and that is absolutely fine. Some women might need the artificial version of oxytocin (syntocinon) because their body is unable to release its own oxytocin due to previous stress or trauma. If they have the insight to know that this is the way they need to birth, own their decisions and take responsibility for their birth experience, it will be a good experience for them. It doesn't make them less of a woman or a bad mother.

Can we compare childbirth to other experiences?
Women often want to find out what the childbirth experience is going to be like, and there are many analogies relating to childbirth, trying to explain or describe what it is like to give birth. Most of them totally miss the most crucial point – that childbirth is a physiological event! Biologically and chemically, a woman in labour is different from a woman who is not in labour. Therefore, you can't compare a woman *not* in labour with a woman who is. If we compare childbirth with a visit to the dentist to have a tooth out, based on it being painful and that someone is going to extract something from our body, we are doing a great injustice to the life-changing event that is childbirth, but also demonstrating a deep lack of understanding of birth physiology. I often hear this as an explanation from doctors and women who have used pain medication during the

birth of their babies. They say: 'You wouldn't go and have a tooth out without pain relief, so why would you have a baby without it?'

Let me make this clear: going to the dentist, taking a seat in his chair, opening your mouth and having a tooth pulled out without pain medication would be plain stupid, unless you were using another technique, such as hypnosis, to manage the pain. This is because you will have no build-up of oxytocin or endorphins, the body's natural painkillers, to help handle the pain, as having a tooth out is not an event that requires these hormones. I guess if you fancied your dentist, you might produce some oxytocin, which would aid a bit towards masking any discomfort felt. Also, your body will most likely have some adrenaline in it as it can be scary to go to the dentist. Lastly, there is no baby to admire at the end of the experience; there will only be a tooth for the tooth fairy. To attempt to compare these two events is absurd! There is nothing physiologically similar at all, and all the focus is on the pain rather than the process. It totally fails to mention the power women feel during childbirth. It makes more sense to use this analogy to demonstrate that if you're in an environment that feels like you're about to have a tooth out when labour starts, your body is not going to be able to produce the hormones necessary for a physiological birth, so you need to move to a place that makes you feel safe.

Some people compare labour and birth with the sea, waves and water. I think this might be more helpful, in the sense that I often notice how a woman breathing through the surges of labour sounds very much like the sea rolling in and flowing out. It is also true that the more you fight the waves, the harder it gets and the more tired you become. You need to relax into it and follow its powerful surges, and it will bring you up to the surface for a breath and a rest. I like the analogy of water, and often think of seaweed, which sways with the force of the waves rolling in and then out again, when I'm with a labouring woman. Women intuitively sway with the rhythmical pulling and pushing of their uterine muscles, and if they are using a birth pool or water during labour, they can easily get into any position, following their body's guidance, as it is easy to move around in water.

I think my favourite, and most accurate, birth analogy is one I have heard many times from different people. Imagine a couple making love in the semi-dark, warm and cosy environment of their home. The oxytocin is flowing and they are breathing rhythmically with the surges of the love hormones. They are working up towards climaxing. Just before this happens, the woman suddenly stops and says to the man, 'I think we need to go to hospital so they can monitor your heart. I'm worried that something is going to go wrong.' They immediately transfer to hospital in an ambulance, the man strapped to a heart monitor. They are now in a brightly lit, cold hospital room with nurses and doctors there, keeping an eye on the man's heart rhythm. They say to him, 'You're fine to continue where you stopped at home.' As if that would be possible! It is very likely that all his oxytocin has been replaced by stress hormones, such as adrenaline and cortisol, which will lead to very obvious problems that will prevent the couple from continuing their lovemaking.

Oxytocin is at its highest level in a woman's body during physiological childbirth, and is also at a high level during orgasm. The environment affects the release of oxytocin, as it is known to be a 'shy' hormone and is more easily released in an environment that is semi-dark, warm and quiet. The place where a couple make a baby is the exact environment that a woman needs to be in to increase her chances of a physiological birth. Making love and having a baby are not the same thing, obviously, but all the same hormones are involved, and that is why some women even experience orgasms during childbirth. A survey of midwives showed that they had witnessed orgasms in about 0.3% of births (Postel, 2013) and Ina May Gaskin once conducted a poll of 151 women, of whom 32 reported having at least one orgasmic birth (Pascali-Bonaro, 2008).

Anything that increases the release of oxytocin, such as nipple stimulation, stroking the woman's body, cuddling and kissing, if the woman feels like it, will usually speed up labour and also make the process more manageable. It is not always easy for a man to be told by his wife in labour to rub her nipples in front of the doula and the midwife – although most men are happy to oblige if they understand the positive impact this will have on the birth of their baby.

Caesarean births

When a baby is born by Caesarean, when labour has already started but for some reason is not progressing as is expected, it is generally referred to as an emergency Caesarean. This can sound very dramatic: when we picture an emergency, we tend to imagine blue lights and people in a hurry. This is not usually the case, and if the baby appears well (according to the continuous monitoring that usually takes place at this point), it can be an hour or so before the actual operation takes place. However, if the baby is showing signs of distress in labour and a Caesarean has to happen immediately, this is usually referred to as a crash Caesarean.

An elective or planned Caesarean can be recommended by a doctor for medical reasons as the safest way for both the baby and the mother to give birth. It is usually planned beforehand and carried out as close to the due date as possible, usually in week thirty-nine of pregnancy. For example, if the baby is not growing well or the woman has developed a pregnancy-related illness, such as pre-eclampsia, an elective Caesarean would be medically advised. An elective Caesarean can also be carried out on the request of the mother, and need not be based on any medical indications for surgery.

Often, there can be a lot of negativity surrounding Caesarean births, and many women want to avoid giving birth in this way. Women who have had Caesareans often feel defensive and want to explain that it wasn't their fault that their birth ended up like this. If the woman has chosen to have a surgical birth, she will usually say it was for the best and that she was advised to go down this route. According to the WHO (World Health Organization), the Caesarean birth rate should be 10–15%: in some cases, for example placenta praevia (a condition in which the placenta is too close to the cervix), the life of the baby and/or the mother are at risk if a vaginal birth is attempted. However, we are seeing Caesarean birth rates increasing dramatically each year across the globe.

There are many reasons why a Caesarean birth is not as beneficial for the baby or the mother as a physiological birth or even a non-physiological vaginal birth, especially when women have elective Caesareans, sometimes as early as week thirty-eight of their pregnancy, when their baby might not be ready to be born. As I discussed earlier, there is still no definite explanation of how labour starts, but some studies have suggested that the baby signals to the mother that she is ready to be born, one event in a chain of events that take place during childbirth. What impact does this have on this baby if this link in the chain is missed out? How about the omission of the maternal foetal ejection reflex? The impact of these two steps being missed out could be considerable, and we don't know yet what effect this may have. I'm sure we will discover more about this in future.

What we do know is that babies born via Caesarean are more likely to develop asthma, as they miss out on the journey through the birth canal. There are several benefits to a baby to being born vaginally. The fluid in the baby's lungs is squeezed out and pressure is created for the first breath. The central nervous system is stimulated and starts to organise itself while huge changes take place in the baby's circulatory system. This doesn't happen in the same way when a baby is born by Caesarean.

Babies born via Caesarean are more likely to be obese (Darmasseelane et al., 2014), which new studies on microbiomes have shown is due to the newborn baby's gut not being colonised by healthy bacteria from the mother when passing through the birth canal (Harman, 2014). A Caesarean birth is too sterile – naturally; it is an operation – and babies born surgically are often not put skin-to-skin immediately with the mother, which can lead to problems establishing breastfeeding – and one of the many risks of formula feeding is an increase in obesity (Armstrong, 2002).

When we talk about Caesarean births, we should be grateful that we have the medical knowledge to carry them out safely, as they can save the lives of both babies and women. However, a Caesarean is major abdominal surgery and the recovery time is usually around six weeks. Pain after the operation may be severe, and future pregnancies and births may be compromised. A woman in labour is full of oxytocin, the love hormone, which will pass through the placental blood to the baby. During an elective Caesarean birth, the baby will miss out on the 'oxytocin high' that is experienced after birth by both mother and baby, especially if the baby is not put skin-to-skin immediately with the mother. However, it is never too late for skin-to-skin contact. This will always produce oxytocin in both the mother and her baby, and should be encouraged as long as it feels comfortable for both.

The impact on women of an unwanted Caesarean can be devastating, and may lead to postnatal depression (PND) or PTSD. She might find it difficult to bond with her new baby, which can have a negative impact on the whole family. For the baby, poor bonding might lead to mental health issues as she grows up.

I think we need to focus on educating women and their partners – but also obstetricians – on the long-term impact that unnecessary Caesareans might have on our population. We should not focus on trying to decrease the rate of Caesareans, but we should focus on improving the environment to support physiological birth in hospitals, and encourage women to birth at home or in birth centres. Midwives no longer receive compulsory training in how to support breech and twin vaginal births, which means that women carrying twins or those whose babies are in the breech position are usually recommended to have a surgical birth. Making this experience part of midwifery training could mean that women have more of a choice of how to give birth under these circumstances.

Natural Caesareans

If a woman needs to have a Caesarean birth, there are many good reasons for looking into having a 'natural' Caesarean. It does sound like a contradiction in terms, but this natural approach to a Caesarean birth was developed by Professor Nick Fisk and his colleagues at Queen Charlotte's and Chelsea Hospital in London (Smith et al., 2008).

Some of the features of a 'natural' Caesarean are:

- The baby can be lifted out slowly and gently over several minutes, which is more similar to a vaginal birth. The parents are also able to discover the sex of their baby themselves.

- This gradual birth of the baby allows time for its chest to be squeezed, helping the fluids to clear from the baby's lungs.
- The head of the mother's bed can be raised and the screen usually in place for the operation can be lowered, enabling the parents to watch their baby be born.
- The baby can be put skin-to-skin with the mother immediately after birth, regulating the baby's breathing and temperature.
- The umbilical cord is left unclamped and intact for longer, giving the baby all the benefits of receiving all the placental blood.

If a mother is planning an elective Caesarean, rather than having an emergency Caesarean, it is easier to organise a natural Caesarean, as most obstetricians are yet to be trained in this relatively new procedure. There are resources available online and even a video on YouTube explaining the procedure ('The natural Caesarean: a woman-centred technique', 2011). It could be argued that you should add this to your birth preferences document but, from experience, I know that it can be a challenge to get all this set up and agreed upon in an emergency. I am hopeful that in the future, most Caesarean births will be 'natural' ones, as there are so many benefits to having as close to a physiological birth as possible.

MAKE IT REAL

You may like to think about, or discuss with your birth partner, the following.

The pros and cons of each form of pain medication you might be offered: it is better to research these during pregnancy and have an idea of which you would consider if needed and which you would rather avoid, than risk making an uninformed or a rushed decision during labour.

Similarly, you may want to research different forms of non-pharmaceutical comfort methods, such as a birth pool, a Transcutaneous Electrical Nerve Stimulation (TENS) machine, hot water bottles, acupuncture/acupressure, hypnobirthing and aromatherapy.

If you know that you will be planning an elective Caesarean birth, you may want to think about your preferences, which may include measures to make the birth gentler or more 'natural'. Speak to your care providers about following the procedures of a gentle Caesarean, which include slowing down the birth, delayed cord clamping, immediate skin-to-skin, dimmed lights and a quiet environment. See https://www.mamanatural.com/gentle-cesarean/ for more ideas.

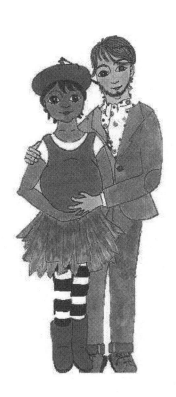

Secret #5:

There is no such thing as perfect parenting — 'good enough' will do.

CR∞

Chapter 5: Being a Mother

There is little that prepares a woman for the massive change a newborn baby will make to her life. It is not unusual for women to have thoughts along the lines of 'What have I done?' or 'I have no life of my own any more' during the days and weeks that follow the arrival of their baby.

I can categorically state that being a mum is the most challenging, tough, guilt-ridden and intense job a woman will ever have! All women understand that things will be different when they have a baby, but I'm pretty sure no one fully realises the immense responsibility they will take on, and how much of themselves they will have to give up.

The majority of new mums may feel overwhelmed and tearful a few days after the birth of their baby. This usually coincides with their milk coming in, and hormones playing havoc with their body. I can still remember how I felt, looking at photos from when my first daughter was born and the day we brought her back from hospital. I'm standing next to the Moses basket where she is lying, and I'm trying to put on a brave smile while my whole body is giving another message and my eyes are red from crying. It all just felt so overwhelming! In the weeks that followed, I felt like I was living in a nightmare with a baby who just cried, fed and cried some more. I can clearly remember putting her down in her cot in the end one afternoon and sitting on the step by the back door, thinking, 'I've ruined my life!' Of course, the next thought that entered my head was how horrible I was for thinking that, and that my daughter had not asked to be born: I had wanted her! It seemed to me that my baby was having a very sad life, crying and being upset all the time. Oh, how I wished I had someone there to tell me that it was absolutely fine to feel how I was feeling, and to reassure me that I wasn't a 'bad' mother and that most mothers feel like this at some point.

Gradually, I started to realise that my baby didn't actually cry all the time, even though it felt like it, and that a baby crying doesn't necessarily mean they are sad or upset; this is the only way babies have to communicate. I learnt to appreciate that if I managed to have a shower, get dressed and go out for a walk I was having a good day. So what if all the washing and ironing didn't get done, or dinner was served later than usual? Going out, meeting other new mums and sharing my experiences with others helped, and I still see many of those mums today. We have been through new challenges as our children have grown up, and parenthood is still hard at times, but I wouldn't change it for the world!

I believe that many women make the early days with their baby more difficult, just like I did, because they want things to get back to 'normal' (i.e., how they were before the baby). Struggling to live the life we used to live before the baby arrived causes us the greatest pain. We are grieving for something that we have lost and that will never return again – because life will never be the same again! Things will eventually return to a state of 'normality', but it will be a new normal, and it will change regularly! The biggest lesson I learnt was to surrender, stop fighting and accept what was happening. The time with a newborn baby is so precious and goes so quickly. Often, new mums wish it away, focused on getting to some point in the future – which is usually the thought of the baby sleeping through the night. But that point in the future doesn't really mean anything. As your child grows up, your concerns change. He will start teething, have colds, have nightmares and night terrors, and when he is eighteen and going to the pub for the first time, most mums will be lying awake, waiting for him to come home, hoping he is safe.

Sleepless nights are part of being a parent, but over time they will happen less often.

Being a mother is a job for life, and the journey a woman takes with her growing child is the greatest and most fulfilling work she will ever do. The memories of funny things your child said when they started talking; the nativity play where your daughter chose to be an angel after telling you, 'I know how much you love angels, Mummy'; and a hug from a teenager who tells you 'I'm so lucky to have you' far outweigh those early days of sleep deprivation and despair.

I believe that the moment a woman can accept that her life is now different, can put aside all thoughts of getting to a mythical 'better' point in the future and simply take one day at a time, the better it will be for her. However, I think that a woman has to be living it and feeling it to get to a place where she is ready to take that step of acceptance. It's not something that you can tell someone to do, and the time it takes will vary from woman to woman. Being a mum is the best and biggest experience a woman will ever have. It comes with ups and downs, but there is nothing that will ever compare to it!

The early days
I'm often saddened by how many new parents worry about the choices they make in looking after their child and their lack of confidence that they are doing the right thing. There are also still many old beliefs around – such as a baby needs to be taught how to self-soothe and you shouldn't respond to a baby every time they cry. It seems as though everyone has totally misunderstood attachment theory, and parents worry that if they pay too much attention to their baby, he will grow up to become so dependent on them that he will never be able to function on his own. Bowlby's evolutionary theory of attachment suggests that babies are born biologically pre-programmed to form attachments with others, because this will help them to survive. The baby is born to demonstrate innate behaviours, called 'social releasers', such as crying and smiling, that stimulate natural caregiving responses from adults.

Bowlby observed that a child would initially form only one primary attachment (monotropy), and that this person acted as a secure base from which the child could explore the world. This attachment relationship becomes the prototype for all future social relationships, so disrupting it can have severe consequences. This theory also suggests that there is a critical period for developing an attachment (from birth to five years). If the child has not developed an attachment to a primary caregiver during this period then he will suffer from what Bowlby believed to be irreversible developmental consequences, such as reduced intelligence and increased aggression (Bowlby, 1958). It appears to be crucial that parents respond to their baby's needs so that the baby can develop the knowledge that he is safe in the world and that his needs are respected and responded to.

The belief that babies need to be left to cry for their own good and to help them become independent is outdated. Research now shows that this could have a negative impact on the emotional development of the child. Babies who are left to cry themselves to sleep have high levels of cortisol in their body even after they seem to have soothed themselves (Middlemiss et al., 2011).

Babies are very dependent on a significant other, which is usually the baby's mother or father, to survive infancy. Human babies are born less able to survive than other baby mammals, as they cannot walk so are unable to follow their parents around, and they can only digest milk, which means they need their food source to be nearby.

What social scientists have recently discovered is that a baby's first three months outside the womb should be thought of as part of the pregnancy trimesters; this time is often referred to as the *fourth trimester*. A baby still needs the cocoon-like environment of the womb to feel snug and warm, and needs to be near the familiar heartbeat which she has associated with comfort and safety. A baby is not born with the cognitive development to understand cause and effect or to be able to manipulate its parents. Babies are wired, very simply, for survival, and their instinctive behaviour is to ensure they get attention when their physical and biological health is threatened. So if they feel too cold or too hot, they will cry. If they feel hungry or unprotected, they will cry. They will feel most settled and happiest in the arms of their parents, close to their familiar smell, heartbeat and voice. I think all new parents should invest in a good sling so they have the option to carry their baby close to them all the time. I recommend a sling, not a baby carrier, as slings are better for your back. There are quite a few different makes and types of slings, including wraps made by Ergobaby and Moby and ring slings such as the Maya sling or the Ellaroo. It's best to try a few out before you buy one, as different slings suit different women. There are many sling libraries popping up in bigger cities, where you can hire a sling before you buy one or instead of buying one. These are excellent for learning more about 'wearing' your baby and what sling suits you best.

A baby is a small human being, and the personality and characteristics that can be observed in a newborn baby can still be observed in that child as she grows up. Babies are not puppies that need to be trained to behave in a certain way – they need their parents to generously give them unconditional love and unwavering support. The expectations new parents have of what a baby should be doing and how they should be behaving are often far from reality. All babies cry – that's how they communicate! When adults cry, it is usually because they are in pain or they are sad, whereas babies cry because they need someone to respond to them. It is important for new mums to understand this, as it can be upsetting to think that your baby is sad all the time, or in pain. It's better to try and imagine that your baby is communicating with you in the only way she is able to.

The first few weeks and months with a new baby can be challenging, but I urge all new parents to try and enjoy this time as much as they can. This time passes so quickly and can never be recaptured. As your baby grows up, becomes a toddler, a teenager and then an adult, you will fondly remember their babyhood. Each stage of a child's life is precious, and it's a shame that many parents look forward to the next stage rather than enjoying the present one and savouring each moment. I can promise that the day your child stops coming into your bed at night after a nightmare – or just because they want to be near you – you will miss it!

Living 'here and now'

Being pregnant and preparing for your upcoming birth and the first few months with your baby can be a worrying time. Increasingly, women are having babies later in life, and by the time they become a mother, they have spent much of their lives studying and building a career. Women use experts to help organise their weddings, to buy a house, to help them look their best and to get fit. There seems to always be someone else who knows more than you do. The thought of getting it wrong with their child makes women pay experts to advise them what to do and how to do it.

For women to take full responsibility for their choices, they need to ensure that they don't blame anyone or anything for the situation they are in – and this also includes themselves. Whether during the birth or postnatally with their baby, women need to accept that each moment is just as it should be. It is easy to struggle against the moment, be unaccepting of what is happening, and wish that the situation – or what is actually happening – was different. It is possible to wish for things to be different in the future, but in this moment, right now, things are as they are.

Most of us react to situations and people's actions around us and we may feel upset, angry or disappointed. For example, as a new mum, you might not get anything else done during the day apart from feeding your baby. This might make you feel fed up and angry that the baby is making your life difficult, and you might look at other mums and think that you must be doing something wrong as they don't seem to have the same problems. These feelings belong to us and we can't blame them on another person or on a situation. When we can see this and recognise that we have a choice over how we react, we are able to take full responsibility for the situation. Challenges or problems give us the opportunity to change and to accept what is. When we meet challenges with resistance and anger, or blame others, our lives become harder. We need to learn to bend and move with challenges, and avoid staying rigid.

Sometimes all we need to do is stop fighting and surrender to the present moment, because the pain we are feeling is the pain of the fight, not the pain of the problem.

When women can experience their birth and parenting in the present and consciously decide to stay here and now, the struggling will stop and she will have an indescribable feeling of peace and calm. The present is the only time that is real. If we can make the most of this moment – treasure it, knowing that it will never come again – we can enjoy it more fully.

Quick fix
Waiting for nine months to meet your baby can seem a long time. Women tend to slow down and become more introverted, focusing on their baby's arrival and wondering what it will be like to be a mother. This time is important, as life with a baby is lived much more slowly – it takes longer to get things done! If women still expect things to be the same with a baby, they are in for a surprise.

The challenges and hurdles that parenthood brings are not as easily dealt with as some of life's other problems. Today, we are all used to finding a quick fix for our problems: we will search the web, ask all our friends for their advice, and spend as much as we can on finding a solution. It is not often that we simply accept that, for now, things are as they are, and in the future, things will most likely change on their own. As strange as it may sound, the more we focus on a problem, the more energy we give it, and it just seems to get bigger and bigger until it seems insurmountable.

A challenge with a baby can take weeks or months to 'solve' – and usually it fixes itself without any need for intervention! The baby grows and develops and what once was an issue, all of a sudden, is no longer an issue. However, there are usually plenty of new hurdles popping up ahead. Being a parent means that there will always be something going on that you wish you could fix or make go away: sleep problems, eating problems, friend problems, school problems, broken hearts, illness, disappointments – the list goes on and on. As a parent, you could live the rest of your life with a sense of failure if you always try to find a solution to everything that you experience with your baby and child. At times, being a parent is an endurance sport. Things will change again, and there will always be something new or different to accept.

Relationships

Having a baby has a huge impact on the new parents. The man may feel that he is no longer as important to his partner as he used to be, and the woman may feel unheard and unsupported. Women often tell me that their partner doesn't understand what an enormous impact having a baby has had on them: in their view, nothing has changed for him and everything has changed for them! The men still go off to work every morning, have their sessions in the gym and go out with their mates for a few beers.

Women often don't want to leave their babies with anyone else, and feel like a lioness with her cub, even unhappy sometimes with the way her partner is holding and handling the baby. I know that men try to offer their help but because they are not caring for the baby exactly as the women are, they often get told off, the woman takes over and the man goes away, thinking he's not very good at this baby stuff. It doesn't need to happen very often for the man to decide to stay away, as he seems to always do it wrong anyway. In his view, the woman is doing a great job, so why not let her get on with it?

Very recently, neurologists have discovered that, even before a woman gives birth, pregnancy changes the structure of her brain. These changes in her brain can be linked to the way the woman acts during pregnancy and also as a new mother. What neurologists have discovered is that activity increases in regions that control empathy, anxiety and social interaction. These changes, brought on by a flood of hormones during pregnancy and after birth, help the mother bond with her baby. In other words, the maternal feelings of overwhelming love, fierce protectiveness and constant worry begin with reactions in the brain. For women, the behaviours of mothering are there in her brain as a blueprint long before she becomes a mother. These changes are most significant when a woman is having her first baby, and it is not clear whether the brain ever goes back to its pre-pregnancy state (Abraham et al., 2014).

On the other hand, men don't have this blueprint or structural change in their brain when becoming fathers. Instead, evolution has created other pathways in the brain for men to adapt to their role as fathers, and this is achieved through practice and day-to-day care of the baby (Abraham et al., 2014).

Biologically and physiologically, women and men become parents differently. If we can be aware of this, I believe we could understand and support each other a lot better and with much more empathy. Women are responding to a hormone-fuelled blueprint of behaviour which, at times, they have no conscious control over, and men can only become good fathers if they get the chance to look after their babies.

I encourage my clients to speak honestly to each other about how they are feeling. It's important to talk using 'I' statements – that is, to say 'I am feeling sad/left out' rather than 'You are making me feel terrible!' Becoming parents is a challenge for both the mother and the father, and it takes a little bit of time to get used to the new normal.

MAKE IT REAL

You may like to think about, or discuss with your birth partner, the following.

Making a self-care plan for once your baby is born. You might want to consider how you will be able to rest as much as possible, what help you may enlist, which foods you would like to nourish you, managing visitors, and setting up a 'nest' where you can snuggle up with your baby and rest and sleep.

What is normal for infant sleep? Knowing what is normal, and yes, I'm talking lots of night waking and frequent night feeds, is very helpful.

If you have a partner, how will you nurture your relationship and each other when you are both exhausted and coming to terms with the wonderful but all-consuming new addition to your family? Within this, you may also want to discuss your expectations around chores and baby care, before the baby is born. Do you both expect the parent on maternity leave to do the chores? Perhaps you feel that you're both 'working' and chores should be shared equally? Or that, during the first few weeks and months, the new mother should do as little as possible to fully recover? Maybe you expect whoever is out at work to take over in the evenings so the parent at home can have a little respite? There is no right answer, only what is right for you.

There are almost as many books and theories about parenting as there are parents! I am not suggesting you go out and buy every book, but having some discussions about how you plan to parent in the early days before your baby arrives could be beneficial to ensure you are on the same page.

She enters her birth as a woman and leaves as a mother.

CREOD

Chapter 6: What Being a Doula has Taught Me

As I look back at the past twelve years and the births I've been privileged to support at, I have come to realise that nothing teaches you about life the way birth does. It is the ultimate challenge for women, when they come face to face with who they truly are. If viewed as a way of providing insight into areas within that could do with some attention, it can lead to the opportunity and freedom to lead a more fulfilling life. Every woman and couple I have supported has taught me something new about myself. I am forever in their debt, and I am so grateful that they let me share this special time with them. I have also witnessed the transformation that takes place in women, their partners and their families when they experience a good birth that they felt fully part of.

There are some births at which I was present that had a greater impact on me and that brought me to a different level – or, rather, triggered a transformation in me, which was further cemented into my being in the births that followed.

If you think about it, childbirth is an event in a woman's life where there is nowhere to hide. It's a forced transformation: she will gain a new identity; she enters her birth as a woman and leaves as a mother. In the process of giving birth to her baby, she is not in control of what is going on in her body, and she cannot change her mind or back out of her commitment to have a baby. Whether she has a Caesarean birth or a vaginal birth, she has been on a journey during her pregnancy in which she has discovered and learnt a lot more about herself, whether she wanted to or not; just by being pregnant and having her body governed by strong hormones and occupied by another living being. She may have had to slow down if she was very active prior to getting pregnant; perhaps pregnancy hormones have made her absent-minded; or maybe she has found her priorities have changed and many things in her life that she used to think were important have suddenly become unimportant.

We are so attached to dichotomies in the world we live in: everything has to be one thing or the other: good or bad, traumatic or ecstatic, beautiful or ugly. If we could accept that things are what they are and that each of us needs to take responsibility for our own actions, feelings and thoughts, I don't think anyone would feel they have 'failed' at birth. If we could look back at what we can learn from our birth experience and also how we can heal from it, we can see every experience as something positive. Our baby's birth might not have been exactly as we hoped it would be, but we can still gain something from it.

It just is what it is!

Now I would like to share with you some stories from my clients, who have taught me so much. I have changed their names and some of the details so that they remain anonymous.

Seema and Nitin

Seema made an initial enquiry before she was even pregnant. She sent me an email, commenting on my website and adding that she and her husband had decided to try for a baby and how did she go about booking me? I wrote back to her to let her know that I thought it was great that she was looking into having the support of a doula for the birth of her baby, but I was unable to book her in as I would need a due date for the baby. To my delight, two months later, I had another email to let me know that she was pregnant.

I met them early on in the pregnancy. Seema and her husband Nitin were a lovely couple and very excited about having a baby. Seema had lost her mum a few years back and felt that she wanted female support for the birth. Her mum had been a midwife and she was missing her a lot. After initially thinking about having the baby at the local hospital and after having visited both the birth centre and delivery suite, Seema decided that she wanted to have her baby at home. The local community midwives were very supportive, and Seema and Nitin were looking forward to the day their baby would arrive.

One Friday, Seema's waters went around 7.30 a.m. She phoned me and was very excited. She told me she had also been having period pains throughout the night. She was going out to do some shopping and had sent Nitin to work for the day. She sounded very positive and chirpy. The midwives came out and checked the baby's heartbeat and the colour of the amniotic fluid, and all was good. That evening I had a call from Nitin asking me to come out, as her contractions seemed quite strong.

I arrived around 8.30 p.m. and could tell that Seema was in the very early stages of labour. I stayed for about an hour and a half and told them that they should go to bed and get some rest. I also told Seema how important it was that she ate well, little and often, and drank lots of water. She was having contractions every six to seven minutes, lasting for about thirty seconds.

I spoke to them on Saturday morning. Everything seemed to have stopped, and even the amniotic fluid had stopped trickling out. I spoke to Seema again that afternoon and suggested that they went out for a meal that evening. The midwives had been in contact and had left a message to say that Seema and Nitin should go to the hospital on Sunday at 8 a.m. to induce the labour, unless things progressed overnight. Seema had also had two phone calls from the hospital asking her to come in to be checked over. Seema told me that she was tired and didn't feel like going in. I ended the conversation, telling her to call me if she wanted me to come over.

I phoned Seema at 7.30 a.m. on Sunday morning. I said that I was going to have a shower, eat breakfast and come over so that we could have a chat. I arrived around at 9 a.m. and I found Seema slumped on the toilet, rocking back and forth. She said that the contractions would not stop; she was experiencing one continuous contraction with no chance to rest. She also said that she couldn't pass urine. Seema did not look well at all, so I said to Nitin that we should call the community midwives to come out to assess her, and perhaps we needed to go into hospital.

The phone rang twenty minutes later. It was the community midwives, who wanted to speak to Seema. They came around half an hour later. Seema was two to three centimetres dilated and, after a discussion with the midwives, Seema and Nitin decided that it would be best to transfer into hospital.

We arrived around 1 p.m. and finally got our assigned midwife at 2 p.m. Seema's contractions were coming every ten minutes and she was still uncomfortable. She was very tired. After having an epidural and being given syntocinon to speed up labour, a catheter was sited and over a litre of urine was drained from her bladder. This made her feel and look a lot better. Nitin went home to sleep, and I promised I would keep him informed of Seema's progress.

Seema was examined at 4 p.m. and was still two to three centimetres dilated. The labour was going well until an epidural top-up, together with an increase in syntocinon, led to the baby's heartbeat dropping alarmingly. The syntocinon drip was stopped. Over the next three contractions, the baby's heartbeat stabilised and after thirty minutes, the baby was happy again. The syntocinon was started again at a lower level. After this, the epidural top-ups were administered differently: Seema was given the drug in two small doses, administered a short time apart. This kept the baby happy. The midwives had a shift change and another examination was carried out at 8.30 p.m., after which Seema told me that she felt like 'her bum was going to explode': she was fully dilated. She had done so well!

I rang Nitin, who returned to the hospital, and the second stage of labour – the pushing stage – started at 9.35 p.m. Seema was finding it difficult to push, as she couldn't feel the contractions, but after some demonstrations and explanations of how and where to push, she was pushing really well.

As the epidural wore off and she could feel the contractions building up, it became easier, and she pushed out a beautiful baby girl at 10.56 p.m. Nitin was in absolute awe, having watched his daughter enter the world, and it took him a while to be able to tell his wife that they had a girl! Seema was so happy to finally meet the person she had carried for nine months.

As I left the hospital and walked around the corner to the car park, I suddenly became very aware of the presence of someone thanking me for looking after Seema. Perhaps it was a lack of sleep that had made me hallucinate, as it had been a very long birth, but to this day I'm sure that it was Seema's mum.

The early stages of labour can be challenging for both the woman and her partner. It is really important to eat and drink regularly to ensure you're well hydrated, as well as having enough energy for labour and birth. A birth experience can still be good even if it is different from what you had hoped for. Meeting your baby for the first time is such a special moment.

Eva and Steve

That story brings me on to another story about a young couple, Eva and Steve, who were having their first baby. Steve had been brought up in a very masculine environment, and demonstrated a clear lack of being in touch with his feminine side. Eva would often complain to him that he didn't show her enough affection or cuddle her when she was sad, and she would often get frustrated with his lack of empathy.

Labour started early one evening, and we all stayed at home the whole night, until Steve couldn't wait any longer. He needed to know if things were progressing and how long it was going to take. We arrived at the birth centre where Eva was planning to have her baby and, on examination, she was found to be two centimetres dilated. She had had eight hours already of regular contractions, and this news was rather frustrating for Eva – but even more so for Steve. He was sitting on the birth ball in the room, bouncing up and down, which really irritated Eva. Eva was saying how difficult it was and that she wasn't sure she would be able to do it any more. Trying to be helpful, Steve pointed out to her that women had been giving birth for thousands of years, so why couldn't she do it? This made Eva cry, and she told him how unhelpful it was for him to try and belittle what she was going through, and that him trying to 'fix' everything was just irritating.

We decided to go back home again to rest and I cooked everyone some breakfast on our return. Eva was getting exhausted and, by now, the TENS machine had been on for so long that she was rocking back and forth with the electric pulses that were being emitted from the small pads stuck onto her back. We tried a combination of positions to help the baby move into a better position. I told Eva that she was doing so well, and that we knew it was really tough for her right now.

When we returned to the birth centre hours later, Eva was found to be seven centimetres dilated – but also totally exhausted, as she had been labouring for over thirty hours. During this time, I had noticed how Steve had changed his approach to Eva and was acknowledging her feelings when she said it was hard: he was telling her how brave and strong she was, and trying very hard to not say the wrong things. I had also seen Eva responding to this in a positive way. This guided Steve, and his confidence grew as he recognised how to empathise with his wife. Eva needed some sleep and took the midwife up on her offer of pethidine and lay down on the bed to get some sleep. As the pethidine was working and Eva was drifting off, I couldn't help but notice the space on the bed behind her. I whispered to Steve to go and lie down next to Eva and cuddle her, while I planned to sit in the chair outside and get some sleep as well.

Around four hours later, Eva woke and got into the pool. Her baby was born after a very long labour, and she did it with sheer determination and willpower. I was in awe of her amazing strength, as I always am with women in labour.

When I met up with them a week later Eva said to me, 'One of my most precious memories of the birth was when I had the pethidine and Steve came and lay behind me, just holding me. It made me feel so supported, and it eased the pain as I felt he took some of it from me. As a child, I used to have ear infections all the time and my mum used to give me painkillers but she never took me into her bed or lay next to me, just holding me. If my child ever has pain or is unwell, that is the first thing I will do – hold them, as I now know what a huge difference it makes.'

It brought tears to my eyes as I thought about Eva as a child and all the other children in the world who are in pain and not being held by anyone. She then said: 'I know it was you who told Steve to do it, so thank you.' Straight away, I turned to Steve and told him that he shouldn't have said anything to Eva, as he could have stored up those brownie points for a very long time, and we all had a good laugh.

I have total faith that women will find this amazing inner strength that they aren't aware of themselves. They usually bring that strength out if they feel listened to and empathised with. If a woman feels heard and given the freedom to 'give up' if she wants to, she usually seems able to turn things around and find the courage to carry on. There is usually no need to 'fix' anything.

Wanda and Neil
Initially, after meeting this couple, I was unsure whether they would hire me as their doula. During our meeting, the husband, Neil, was looking as though he was falling asleep and I wasn't sure that I connected with his wife, Wanda. Nevertheless, they wanted me to be their doula and I thought that, as we got to know each other, it would all fall into place.

As with all clients, I planned to have at least two antenatal sessions with them. I noticed in both these sessions that Wanda seemed preoccupied. On one occasion, as we were sitting down to talk, her food shopping arrived and after putting it away, she told me that she was feeling rather tired, so was going to have a rest. I was beginning to think that perhaps I wasn't the right doula for them.

I started my on-call period with them, which for doulas is usually two weeks before the due date. About a week into this, I had a phone call just after midnight from Neil. I could hear Wanda hyperventilating in the background, and Neil was saying, 'I don't know what's going on, but Wanda is having some kind of...', and I could hear Wanda in the background saying, 'Physical reaction'. I asked Neil to hand the phone over to Wanda and I talked her through how to slow her breathing down, reassuring her that everything was all right. As she calmed down, she said that the baby had kicked out and this had caused a panic attack. Wanda was worried that there was something wrong, so I told her to ring the hospital and see what they thought. We agreed to speak in the morning, and I put the phone down.

The next morning, I spoke to Wanda, and she told me that they had decided to go into hospital just to be checked over – and everything had been fine. By now, I was thinking that this was one of the strangest experiences I had ever had. I just couldn't put my finger on what was going on.

A week after the due date, I got a call out of the blue from Wanda. She said to me, 'Kicki, my therapist has told me that I should share something with you. I was sexually abused as a child, and I wanted you to know.' All the pieces suddenly fell into place and I replied, 'I'm so sorry to hear that happened to you. That should not happen to anyone. Thank you for sharing this with me.' Wanda said goodbye and I just stood there, holding the phone, feeling terrible for having been so preoccupied with how *I* had been feeling about the whole situation instead of really focusing on Wanda. We never talked about the abuse again.

That evening, Wanda started labour in her bedroom. She lay on her side, in her bed, and this is where she stayed the whole time. She was writing down every contraction in a notebook, using a small battery-operated fan to cool herself down, and she did not want me or Neil in the room when she had a contraction. In between, we could come in to check on her and bring water and snacks. After a few hours, Wanda called me in and said, 'I think I'm nine centimetres now, perhaps we should go to the hospital?' I asked her if she wasn't getting tired of keeping track of the contractions and writing them down in her book; I thought that she was not in labour since her behaviour was very neocortex-driven. Wanda said that she was getting a bit tired, but she was sure her calculations were right in terms of how far along she was. (She was using the NICE guidelines that the cervix should be dilating one centimetre per hour in labour. These have now been updated to one centimetre every two hours.)

Neil helped her to the bathroom and we then set off on the short trip to the hospital. On arrival, we were met by a lovely midwife and, on examination, Wanda was found to be nine centimetres dilated, just as she had predicted. The second stage of labour was very difficult for Wanda, but after trying many positions and with the very gentle loving touch of her husband, she finally gave birth to her beautiful baby. Wanda turned to Neil and proclaimed, 'I did it!' – and she most certainly did! It was such a lovely and healing experience for Wanda, and I felt so blessed to have been part of her journey.

People are the way they are for a reason, and often we don't have the patience or awareness to look beyond what someone is allowing us to see. The day a woman births her baby is not just another day in her life, it's the accumulation of all her previous experiences. On a subconscious level, women sometimes stop themselves from going into labour because there is something about the experience that they are fearful about. Women often simply need the space to feel safe enough to share some of those fears. Birth can be a healing experience once you feel brave enough to let go into the process.

Giving birth
is so interwoven
with the identity
of being a woman
that it's not
surprising that
it can alter a
woman's self-image.

☙❧

Chapter 7: Birth Stories

It can be very comforting and heart-warming to read birth stories when we are pregnant and preparing for our own baby's birth-day. These stories that some of my clients – and friends – very kindly wanted to share with you are included here to encourage and inspire you for your upcoming birth. There are a variety of stories, and none are right or wrong: rather, each story is unique. Birth can be challenging at times, and hard, but in the UK and other developed countries it is very rarely dangerous. What you will read about here is how these women took away something from their birth, and how their experiences changed them as people.

Catherine's story

We found out we were expecting twins only about seven weeks into my pregnancy. Seeing those *two* little blobs on the ultrasound screen was magical and, from that moment, I was in love and focused on doing everything I could to nurture them and keep them safe.

At thirty-seven weeks, I went into the Outpatients department for a routine check-up and ended up being admitted with suspected pre-eclampsia. The ward was crowded, very hot and full of women being induced and in the early stages of labour. I'm glad that I didn't know then that it would be my home for the next five days!

I didn't have any fixed ideas about whether I wanted a natural birth or a Caesarean. Somehow, despite getting to thirty-seven weeks with twins, I hadn't really thought about the birth, made a birth plan or even packed a hospital bag! In the end, the decision was taken out of my hands, and I was strongly advised to have a Caesarean as James, the bottom twin, was stubbornly in the breech position.

Over the next five days, the babies and I were closely monitored while we waited for a slot to become available for a Caesarean. The women in the beds around me came and went and time ground to a halt – I began to think these babies were never coming and I was destined to be a giant struggling beached whale for ever! When the big day finally arrived, the midwife came to collect us and told my husband to bring two nappies and two hats to the operating theatre. That really brought it home to me that we would be leaving the theatre with two brand new people.

The epidural worked very well and it was an odd feeling to be lying there awake with no pain but with the feeling somebody was washing up in my stomach! Then suddenly I heard the most beautiful sound I had ever heard – the cries of our newborn son, James. After the longest minute of my life, I heard the equally wonderful sound of Finlay's cries.

Unfortunately, I lost a lot of blood during the operation and so began to feel quite ill (I later had to have two blood transfusions). The midwife brought James to me and I remember feeling quite strongly that they should take him away and give him to my husband to look after while I focused on getting through the operation. That was quite an odd feeling, as I had always imagined that when meeting my baby for the first time I would be overwhelmed with love and want to hold him. Instead, all that came later, in the recovery room, where I was able to hold both my babies, try to feed them, and marvel at our two precious little miracles.

I stayed in hospital with my twins for five days. I found the recovery – and trying to care for and breastfeed the babies – exhausting, difficult and overwhelming. The ward was full, the staff were overstretched, and there was very little help available after visiting hours, when the twins' adoring father and grandmother were sent home. We were delighted when we were finally discharged, and from the moment we got home things became easier and easier. That was over a year ago and it's now hard to believe that our bouncing, boisterous toddlers were so tiny and helpless!

Since the birth of my gorgeous boys, I have been lucky enough to spend time with doulas and my eyes have really been opened to how I could have empowered myself to have a more positive birth experience. Do I have any regrets? No. It was still the best day of my life because my boys were born healthy and perfect. Would I do things differently if we are lucky enough to have another go? Yes. I will approach the experience armed with knowledge, experience and far more awareness of my choices.

My birth story is just the first chapter in the magical story of my sons' lives, and being part of that story as it unfolds is a true joy and privilege.

Miranda's story
I was due to give birth for the first time on the 22nd December, 2012. I was quite nervous about it. Not only is it a major life event, but as soon as people find out you're expecting, they happily pass on their words of wisdom ('It's called labour for a reason, because it's hard work. But you get a beautiful little baby at the end of it') or their 'war stories' of long, painful births which generally end with some sort of medical intervention. At the end of the day, I knew that I would have to go through it.

At our NCT classes we had talked through all the pain relief options and the advantages and disadvantages of each. I was very keen to try to do it as naturally as possible, for multiple reasons, ranging from the health of the baby to the fact that I really dislike needles and anything medical. I really did not want have to have a Caesarean, or epidural, but I also knew that the best-laid plans often don't work out, so I wasn't going to beat myself up if I did need medical help. I was booked into the birth centre, so was hoping I'd be able to have a water birth. My sister had given me a book called *Birth Skills*, which ran through all the different coping mechanisms you can use during labour, such as breathing, vocalising, squeezing stress balls, warm water, etc.

One couple at our NCT group had done a hypnobirthing course and passed around *The Hypnobirthing Book* by Katherine Graves. My partner, Graham, read the first couple of pages which really resonated with him, so he was keen to find out more. There wasn't a hypnobirthing course before our due date, but we managed to get a copy of the book. I read about half of it, and a few things really stuck with me: primarily, the fact that women have been giving birth naturally for thousands of years and our bodies are built for the task. The book also helped me to understand what my muscles would be doing during the birth. The sides of the uterus were pulling up, to open up the cervix, and then, when the time was right, pushing the baby down to the birth canal. Simple!

I'm also a firm believer in positive thinking, and because I was fairly anxious about what giving birth was going to be like, I found myself reading the positive birth statements in the book, which I felt would help to block out the 'war stories' I'd heard. I only read them about three or four times, each time just before I went to sleep, so the statements were the last thing I saw. After them, I always had positive dreams and woke up excited about meeting our baby, rather than anxious about giving birth.

My due date came. I was feeling good, with no twinges, so I thought our bundle of joy wouldn't be arriving for a while. The next morning Graham and I were lying in bed reading the papers when I started to feel something like period pains. When I went to the loo, it was a bit gunky and bloody. I remember saying to him, 'I think the party is starting.' My mum was staying with us at the time, and I'm not sure why, but I didn't want to say anything to either of them to cause a fuss. I was feeling particularly private and didn't want to feel that I was being watched.

As the day went on the aches were increasing, but we managed to walk to a local café for a late lunch. I was a bit quiet. I remember walking home at about 4 p.m. very slowly and steadily while my mum and Graham chatted, stopping to look at houses and birds on the way. When I got home I put a film on and sat with my back against the radiator. By about 5 p.m., it was obvious I was having contractions. I recalled from the books and classes that the surges (or contractions) should be forty to sixty seconds long before you go to hospital. I was keen to wait until this point, because I really didn't want to go through all the hassle of getting a cab to hospital and being told to go home again.

By 6.30 p.m. I asked Graham to put the TENS machine on my back. It actually helped a lot. It seemed to dissipate the pain and I was able to control it. The funny thing was, I wasn't sure how painful it was going to get, so I kept it as low as possible, in order that I could increase the power at a later stage.

At about 8 p.m. I was lying on our bed, just trying to get through each contraction, which seemed to be coming in waves of three. I think I was grunting or squealing quite a lot, but I didn't really care. Graham called a cab and my mum was checking on me when suddenly during one contraction I felt a pop and a gush of water go everywhere. After that I felt the urge to push. I recall saying to Mum and Graham, 'I don't need a cab, I need a fu**ing medic. I'm gonna have this baby here!' But I also knew I wanted to have it in hospital, particularly as we weren't prepared at all at home. Even though the thought of sitting in a cab, stuck in traffic, worried me, I knew I had to get through it. The cab ride was like something out of a movie: the driver jumped red lights while I squealed in the back.

When we got to the hospital, we got to the assessment centre and I gave my name before lying down on the floor to have a contraction. The nurses asked if I could pee in a pot and I thought, 'Are you kidding me? I'm having a baby.' After a few minutes they examined me and found I was nine centimetres dilated. I thought, 'See, I wasn't joking.' They put me in a wheelchair, which was uncomfortable, and took me to the delivery floor. Unfortunately, no birth-pool rooms or normal rooms were available, so they put us in a spare room. To be honest, at that point I would have been happy anywhere I could lie down.

I got on the bed and continued as I had at home, lying on my left side and squeezing Graham's hand. I was told to breathe the gas and air by a rather bossy midwife who said I was breathing too shallowly and the baby would need oxygen. But I had no idea what to do. Thankfully, it was the end of her shift and then we got a lovely young midwife who told me to keep breathing through the tube during each contraction until the pain had gone. Although I was initially cautious, the gas really helped.

It took another couple of hours of contractions before I was ready to push, but time flies when you're concentrating on getting through each one. The contractions seemed to change and it felt like my muscles were pushing down. I knew Graham and the midwife could see the head, so I knew it wouldn't be much longer. During that time I remember the midwife pouring warm water over me 'down there', which felt really nice. It was a big push to get the head out, after which I needed to rest for a few minutes. When my body was ready, I managed one big push and finally this crying, slippery, bloody bundle of joy was placed on my stomach. It was 10.55 p.m. We had a few minutes of tears and elation before we lifted the baby up to discover it was a girl.

The midwife had read my birth plan and didn't ask Graham to cut the cord until it had stopped pulsing. Then I needed to push out the placenta, as I had requested not to have the drug used to speed up the placenta delivery (syntometrine), so the midwife helped me to kneel and push again, while Graham held the baby. It only seemed to take a couple of minutes, and I was lying back with my baby.

Our baby started to suckle within about half an hour of being born, and although the sensation was strange, it wasn't painful.

I had to have a few stitches, as I had torn, which sounds a lot worse than it is, as you really don't notice it at the time. The stitches were a little painful, but I was on such a high with my baby lying on my chest that I managed to get through them.

As her father passed out on the bed beside mine, I lay there staring in wonder at this tiny little girl, who was dozing and suckling. Funnily enough, as I write this over four months on, she is still dozing and suckling – and I am still staring in wonder.

Looking back, I wouldn't have done anything differently. It was one of the most amazing experiences of my life, and I feel incredibly proud of myself, and my body, for getting through it.

Jo's story

I always thought I would have an elective Caesarean. I was originally put off birthing vaginally by an enormous fear of completely ruining my genitals and, consequently, my sex life. I generally disliked going to hospitals to see doctors, or having appointments with the dentist. I particularly hated it when medical professionals treated me with arrogance, impatience, condescension and disrespect, all of which I had experienced during previous treatments for illness.

Above all, it was not the hard-working muscle pain of labour and birth, but a loss of all autonomy, all privacy and all dignity, that I feared the most. I also feared that my husband would feel revulsion at seeing me in a completely undignified, petrified and helpless state. But there was also another, arguably more positive, choice that I had been sure for a long time that I would make if I were pregnant – and that was to hire a doula.

I had read about having a doula many years before in an article in *The Sunday Times*. It sounded like a fantastic and sensible idea: a professional, experienced birth partner, who knew and understood a great deal about pregnancy, birth and early parenthood, who would provide me with personalised, continuous, non-judgemental, emotional and practical support throughout my pregnancy, my labour and birth, and in the weeks beyond. I had been let down by family and friends at difficult times of my life before. I had thought at times that I could rely on them to give me continuous support and understanding but, in the end, their own experiences and strong, judgemental opinions frequently came to the fore. This, coupled with a lack of knowledge of my personal circumstances, meant I had not been given the support I needed.

I interviewed several doulas in order to find the one I had the best connection with. The woman I chose was a newly trained doula who had supported at four births. My husband and I just knew she was the one for us.

I fully explained all my fears to my doula, Emma, and told her that I wanted to be in my own sanctuary and to have quiet, calm and familiar surroundings to labour and birth in. She gave me great information and ideas about where to start, and I began to do some research into how to have a birth that would be the most positive and safest for me as an individual. I quickly found that a home birth not only provided the best birth environment for me, but would also statistically be the safest way for me to birth my baby.

I loved the continuity of care that came with the home birth. Yet it was much more than that: I received encouragement, support, belief, trust and empowerment from both my doula and independent midwife. My local hospital is around ten minutes away, so I felt confident that I could get there very quickly if I had to. I trusted that my experienced caregivers would identify and deal with any issues as they arose during the long hours of labour, and suggest changes of plan if necessary, before any issue became an emergency.

In the end, by the time I gave birth, my strong rapport with my doula and midwives had completely dispelled my original fears of loss of autonomy and dignity.

I had been having cramp-like pains and twinges for about a week before my waters broke, but I just took them to be my body gearing up for labour and I carried on as normal. My due date came and went, so I had two sessions of acupuncture. I explained – truthfully – that I felt I could be subconsciously holding on to the baby due to fear of the enormous change it would bring to my life.

My labour started twelve hours later. I didn't want to get too excited in case I had many hours of labour ahead, and I didn't want to wake Adam unnecessarily, so I went upstairs and listened to my natal hypnotherapy CD for three hours.

By about 8 a.m., I couldn't listen to my CD unless I was on all fours, swaying, and I was finding it hard to consider the cramps just as 'opening sensations' – as they are described on the CD. I went to wake Adam, who complained that I was cold to touch and it was 'too early on a Saturday!' until he realised the reason for waking him. He soon jumped to attention and rang Emma, the doula, and Michelle, the midwife. Emma was round by 10 a.m. and Michelle planned to come later.

From 8.30 a.m. until noon, things progressed really well, although I kept insisting that Emma was only saying that to keep me going!

I used my TENS machine while kneeling on all fours, and swayed and breathed through each contraction. Emma was great. She knew exactly where to rub my back and encouraged Adam to do the same. She asked Adam to leave the room to fill the pool, and she gave me confidence that I would be progressing well. I trusted her completely when she reassured me that it was now time for the pool.

Getting into the pool was absolutely fantastic! I had had a very hot shower about 8.30 a.m., which helped at the time, but feeling the hot water envelop me and cocoon me was a wonderful relief. It helped invaluably in keeping me calm and relaxed. Emma put the music-only version of my natal hypnotherapy CD on in the background and drew the curtains, as well as lighting the scented candles which I had always burnt while listening to the hypnotherapy CD. My mind remembered all the hypnotherapy words from simply hearing the music, and I 'went inside my head' for a large part of the next two hours, taking each contraction at a time. I would breathe in as each contraction came, but then focus massively on breathing out and through the remainder of each contraction, adopting whatever position under the water felt best at the time. In between contractions I would rest in the lovely warm water, conserving my energy and focusing on the music.

I went to the bathroom a couple of times, and it was so nice to be in my own private bathroom at home. I had contractions in the bathroom too, but it was easy to stay focused in the familiar environment, and each time I got out of the pool it felt amazing again when I got back in.

I asked Adam to wait upstairs at this stage with Kate, a good friend of mine, because I wanted to make raw and instinctive physical effort noises, and I felt that I couldn't completely let go and do that in front of him.

Michelle then did an internal examination, which was quick, painless and dignified as it was done under the water, and she delightedly told me that the baby's head was at the top of the birth canal. It was at that point that I remember thinking, 'God, this is really hard now. If I have another twenty hours or so of this, I may have made a mistake about not having an epidural!'

Pushing in the pool was brilliant. I was kneeling or on all fours in the water, and it was very dignified. I began experiencing stronger and stronger expelling contractions, and I found that standing up and kneeling on the side of the pool and doing very fast squats helped to relax me through the contraction, and allowed gravity to help with pushing.

After about forty minutes of hard, but satisfying, pushing, I knew the baby's head was about to be born. Michelle ran to get Adam, who was already on his way back, and as Adam reached me at the side of the pool I birthed the baby's head, so Adam was able to see our baby entering the world.

I birthed my baby in a wide squatting position halfway out of the water, which was very comfortable for me. As a result of being able to go at my own pace and push only when my body wanted to, the baby's head descended and birthed very gently and I had no tearing at all. This is even more amazing as Bob turned out to weigh 10 pounds 2 ounces. It took a few more contractions for the rest of the baby's body to be born.

I held my baby tightly in my arms and was so unbelievably delighted to have him here. A quick glance also confirmed what I had known in my heart all the way through my pregnancy – that it was a little boy; it was our Bob, here to be with us at last.

Michelle and Emma got Adam and me into pyjamas, changed our bed and tucked us in, with Bob on my chest, where he crept up and latched on immediately for his first breastfeed. Michelle and Emma left soon after, with reassuring promises to return the next morning.

Adam and I ordered takeaway pizza and stayed up, dozing on and off, until midnight, gazing at our beautiful son. We felt so lucky to have had such a brilliant physiological birth experience. Adam told the midwife later that the whole experience had been 'surprisingly routine', with no drama, chaos, screaming or difficult, awkward scenes. It was simply relaxed, steady, natural and positive, which is all we had wanted. It has served as a fantastic foundation for the exhausting, rewarding work of being new parents.

Put simply, birthing my son changed my life. Prior to having Bob, I was a full-time barrister. Complex last-minute cases, featuring a number of highly vulnerable persons and their heightened, distressed emotions, were a daily part of my adrenaline-fuelled life. I frequently felt anxious and was my own harshest critic. I strove to remain constantly in control of everything, while holding myself up to constant judgement from myself and from all outsiders.

When Bob was born, I felt an exhilaration and feeling of empowerment that I had never known before. I felt as though I had touched the very edge of life and come out the other side. I felt as though I could do anything, and my near-constant worries about what others (especially family and colleagues) thought of my every act began to fall away. I felt a profound and instinctive attachment to Bob, which grew as I mothered him through breastfeeding.

I now talk to midwives, doulas, doctors and other professionals about human rights in childbirth law, on behalf of Birthrights, and I am a trustee and the Director of Leaders of La Leche League GB, for whom I also do other work globally. When I speak to a group of people about birth and breastfeeding, I often end my talk with a photograph of myself, having just birthed Bob, and with my midwife and doula in the room beside me. I tell them that the support I had when birthing ensured that birthing was transformative for me, and that my doula and midwife are the reasons I now do what I do.

I have come to believe that we should never underestimate the enormous effect of truly being with, and listening to, a birthing woman. Empowering her can utterly transform her view of herself, her relationships with others, and can ultimately have an effect on the lives of all others to whom she then reaches out.

Elsa's story

When I was pregnant with our daughter Lovisa, I read a lot of books. I read everything I could get hold of on pregnancy and labour and early childhood. Yet all the books I came across on labour seemed to start from the point of view that a woman uninitiated in the secrets of labour must be terrified. Every one of the books started from the vantage point that labour would inevitably be painful, and went on to offer 'secrets' or 'strategies' for coping with the trauma of giving birth.

I have never been scared of labour. My mother described her labour with me with predictably revisionist rose-coloured glasses. When pushed, she'd say it was like bad constipation. And I was often told how my parents spent early labour in the park eating marmite sandwiches. I was excited about labour. And as my pregnancy progressed, I came to an understanding about natural childbirth that was quite separate from the idea of having a baby. I wanted to be able to achieve a natural birth as a rite of passage, as an experience that was just for me.

As I was to be a first-time mum, had one miscarriage behind me, and because my husband and I lived and worked in different cities for work, we decided to have our antenatal care and labour under the care of a private OB/GYN. He was a really great and personable man, but as time progressed we found ourselves at odds with regard to our views on labour. In all fairness, his views were probably influenced in part by terrified women, but he in turn was terrified or mistrustful of a non-medical birth.

As I started doing research and considering my options for giving birth, I became familiar with the battleground between OB/GYN-led care and midwifery. I looked longingly at natural birthing centres around London but then become concerned about their lack of medical resources, if they became necessary. I imagined the ambulance ride across town, the transfer and the risks. I thought I would labour best in an environment where I knew help was at hand if needed, so glumly returned to my chosen route of care.

Alongside my OB/GYN, we hired a doula. We bonded immediately. She was calm, grounded and had a great sense of humour. I knew straight off that she was someone I wanted with me. We shared not only the same vision regarding birth, but also the same nationality. It felt destined that we should meet, and she lent me resource after resource. More importantly, she felt like the perfect antidote to the more medically focused world of my appointed consultant. She was my backbone in a world that was still unfamiliar to me.

While my visits to my OB/GYN's offices were always pleasant, tensions slowly mounted. I found myself spending much of the precious time I should be focusing on completing my PhD digging through medical journals in order to appear at his office, triumphant, with counter-evidence at hand. Initially I thought of it as playful banter, but as the big day drew nearer, I started to become unsure.

He put it to me: 'If I needed to have heart surgery, I'd look up the best surgeon in the area, and then I'd just let him get on with it.' I left his office feeling guilty, thinking, 'I'm a troublesome patient: it's not fair on either of us. I should just trust him.' But then I had a realisation. Antenatal care is not like heart surgery. It is fundamentally different. A medically perfect heart operation is a success. Birth isn't like that. Sure, the end goal is a healthy baby. But for most women – and definitely me – the journey is physically and spiritually important too. The most perfect medical birth might still leave me unhappy, unsatisfied and unfulfilled. I longed for a particular birth and, everything being well, I wanted to feel that I had the support necessary to achieve that birth.

I started to feel like no woman who is approaching forty weeks should feel: as if the choices we were making would lead me to the highly interventionist birth I was trying so hard to avoid.

***

I am a few days past my due date when early labour begins. Despite all the advice to the contrary, I'm too excited to go back to sleep. When morning comes, my contractions have slowed and I realise things won't happen as fast as I had hoped. I try to eat and rest, but it's still too much to sleep through. In the evening, things pick up again and my doula arrives. I'm frustrated by the contractions and I'm eager to get going, but I still feel like I am play-acting labour. I keep asking my doula if it is going to get worse and whether we should go in. Eventually, in the middle of the night, we decide to make the trip. We've called ahead, as I want to use a pool, and received the surprising answer that while there are birth pools available, there are no staff in the private ward trained to use them, so first we will go to the birth centre, where they do have pools and staff, and our consultant will meet us there. We're confused but decide to go along with that.

When we arrive I am only two centimetres dilated. We are told we can stay but I might be more comfortable at home. We decide to take a break. Our doula drops us home and goes for a rest. Everyone is telling me to sleep, but the pain makes that impossible. I have to keep moving. I use my husband's pull-up bars to hang from the doorframe, and find that gives the most relief. But the truth is, I want to be in hospital. I want to be where I'm going to give birth. I can't get into the groove until I'm in place. We call the hospital. They say to come back. I'm open to about five centimetres. We stay.

The midwifery birth unit is lovely. I don't know how long it takes, but suddenly I just know that I'm not moving. My birth plan is standard practice here. There are no more arguments. Everyone is on the same page. My consultant pops by and, rather surprisingly, states that he can't assist me in water. He gives me the option to stay, and we decide to transfer out of his care and stay with the NHS.

It's a long day. Our daughter is in an awkward position. But, more than that, I am still struggling to really let go. My mind is micro-managing everything. By mid-afternoon I start to pick up on a sense of concern in the room. Things are clearly progressing too slowly. I get the feeling that, if I don't get my act together, some form of intervention might be necessary.

Everyone tries to keep the concerns about slow progress from worrying me, but I start to realise that I am going to have to take action. I remember thinking, 'Something has to change or I am on a trajectory to the kind of birth I don't want. I realise this is my chance to do this and it will not last forever.' With that, everything clicks into place. Curling up in hot water trying to avoid pain is not going to get me anywhere; it is the pain that will get me where I want to get to. I get out of the pool. The midwife breaks my waters.

I realise that the tension I have always felt between mind and body, growing up with an eating disorder, is what is stopping me. I have to truly trust. I have to let go. I have to let my body do what it has to do.

Within minutes of thinking that, I am on my way into an unreachable place where there is no pain. This state gets deeper and deeper and for the second stage I feel no pain whatsoever.

I sit on a birthing stool with my husband behind me, stimulating my nipples to increase contractions. My midwife tells me when to push. I haven't slept for nearly forty hours at this point so I need to conserve my energy. My doula wafts clary sage through the room, wipes my forehead and encourages me. I am aware of them all, but I'm totally inside myself. Nothing exists but me in this state of extremely focused labour. That's all I am now. I have no other thoughts. I feel nothing, but also everything. I have never been more focused in body and mind. It is like the deepest state of meditation. I feel totally secure, totally confident and so strong.

When my daughter is born it is half past nine in the evening. The room is dark, with only one small light. The mood in the room is elated. The midwife and my doula talk about her masses of hair as she crowns. Do I want to feel the head? I refuse to leave my zone; don't want to do anything to lose focus, so I stay in my elated state, thinking, 'Oh, that's my perineum tearing,' but not feeling any pain whatsoever. Then my midwife tells me that she is going to count to three. On three I will collapse forward onto my knees. I am so exhausted that her firm directions are more than helpful. She counts. I fall forward. My daughter is born moments after. The midwife passes her up to me and I slump back on the cushions with her on my chest. Nothing exists but her, and her calm face. I tell her how amazing she is. How hard she worked. That she's here now. That we did it!

When I look back on my labour, it is forever linked to my deep love for, and the close relationship I have with, my daughter. I feel proud to have achieved the labour I did, but when I think of it now it was not only for me, not just an experience for me, but also built the foundation for how I would be as a mother. I had no idea how I would feel or what I would think about motherhood; what type of mother I would become. Having such a fantastic labour has made me forever confident and proud to trust my body and my instincts. It has finally brought me to a place where I love my body: my body that gave birth, my body that produced glorious (much revered) milk, which has been such a source of comfort and continuity for my daughter over the first three and a half years of her life.

After giving birth to Lovisa and looking back on my pregnancy, and all the books I read that spoke of pain and fear and various strategies to cope, I am reminded of something. I once did a skydive outside Meribel in Switzerland. I'm scared of planes. Nobody spoke much English. I had to sign some liability waiver forms before I jumped. I was terrified. But as soon as the plane was behind me and I was falling, I was in heaven. There was nothing to do but to trust. When I landed, only one thing passed through my mind: I want to do it again.

Alina's story
This is for my mother – who didn't get to have the birth experiences she deserved.

Freya is now two and a half years old and a beautiful, caring and generous spirit. I feel blessed and humbled that she loves me, that she seeks out my company to play with, to chatter to and to give me unsolicited hugs with the comment, 'Mummy, you're my darling.'

For many years I tried not to think about the undeniable fact that, if we were to have children, it would be my body that would change, my body that would bear the battle scars of nurturing a life, and my body that would have to painfully eject this new soul into the world. It seemed grossly unfair that, because I was female, this burden would be mine alone. I pretty much viewed the whole process as something akin to the final scene in Ridley Scott's *Alien*, where a foreign object bursts out of Sigourney Weaver's chest. It used to bug me that when watching childbirth on telly, my husband would tear up because he thought childbirth was so amazing, while I would be sitting there with my face scrunched up and my legs crossed, listening to the moans and cries of pain coming out of the box.

Today I look at my 'battle scars' and wear them with pride. Each silvery stretch mark is a latticework of love – a permanent tattoo of the enduring commitment I have to my daughter. This tattoo is absolutely unique to my body. I feel lucky that I have this lifelong reminder of how amazing my body is – it knows exactly what to do, no matter what my conscious mind says or thinks.

During pregnancy I was surprised by how easy it was and how healthy I felt. It gave me the freedom and responsibility to truly listen to what my body was telling me. I started to feel more confident in being a woman and a lot more powerful because of the incredible way my body was building a life – with or without my conscious involvement. I was fascinated and in love with my changing shape.

My husband Mark and I went to NCT birthing classes. Here we learnt about the mechanics of what happens. The NCT had a very strong message on the contraindications of pain relief. I had always joked that I paid my hard-won wages into my National Insurance, and thus expected the best drugs that money could buy! However, I started to do some exploration online about what birthing experiences I might be able to have with a little bit of support and preparation. And that's when I came across the word 'doula'. 'What a brilliant word,' I thought. As a foreigner with a limited female network in the UK, I wanted a mother's friend: a helper, someone there to coach us into being the best birthing partners we could be. I had also talked to Mark's grandmother, who gave birth at home in London during the Second World War, with only an experienced neighbour helping her. I read how experienced women support birthing mothers in other countries. It seemed to me that there was strength to be found in having women around you during labour.

So I contacted a few doulas. I wanted someone to understand my fears, and to talk through what to expect from a practical point of view. When I met Kicki, I knew instantly that she was absolutely going to be guided by my agenda and that she could support me both from a scientific and psychological point of view. In our very first meeting she eased my concerns and helped me to trust that my body had amazing potential if I just worked with it rather than against it.

Leading up to the birth, Mark and I attended hypnobirthing classes and I started to get very excited at the thought of seeing the love in my husband's eyes as he looked into his daughter's eyes for the very first time. My local health food store and Kicki suggested homeopathic remedies to help bring on labour and help throughout the labouring process. I discussed with Kicki the benefits of a home birth, and knew that I definitely wanted a water birth. In fact, my hypnobirthing meditations all centred on breathing through the strong crashing of ocean waves – something that other people had described the waves of labour as being similar to.

After talking with Kicki, I produced a birthing plan that included the kind of language to be used during my labour. I didn't want people referring to levels of 'pain'; I didn't want bright lights; I didn't want lots of checking to 'see how far along I was'. I just wanted to be left alone to get on with what my body knew it needed to do. Mark was to deal with any questions so I could become introspective, listen to my body and not be distracted. Kicki knew that though I might ask for pain relief (especially during the transition stage), in fact I wanted her to encourage me to wait a bit. These were the things I could control, when most other things were out of my control.

At 1.30 a.m. on 17th February I woke up needing to use the bathroom. 'Hmmm,' I thought, 'either this is an Olympic-winning pee, or my waters have broken.' I had strict instructions from my midwife to call the hospital as soon as my waters had broken, but I knew that if I called, they would ask me to come in, and more than likely I would be sent home again to wait things out. So I had a lovely long shower instead, got my things ready, rang a dear friend in Canada who had given birth to four children, and woke my husband up at 4 a.m.

By now I was experiencing some mild period-type pains, so we were pretty calm. However, the pain soon ramped up and at 5.30 a.m. I rang the hospital, let them know that I wanted a water birth, and checked that there were birth pools free for me to use. Before I got in the car, we attached the TENS machine we had hired. Using that took my mind off what seemed like an interminably long drive (over way too many speed humps) to the hospital.

We were placed in a room and our first midwife examined me. She cheerfully told me I was zero centimetres dilated and to go home. I couldn't believe that it felt this intense already and I hadn't even begun to dilate. I turned to my husband and said, 'I don't care if I have this baby in the car park; I am not getting back in the car again.' Fortunately, the hospital was pretty quiet, and we were allowed to stay in the room once the midwife saw how adamant I was. I leant over the side of the bed and rocked my hips to and fro through each tightening of my belly. Not too long after, I vomited. I remember Kicki telling me that anything like vomiting, singing or making sounds that kept the mouth open was my body's way of helping everything to relax and open up. At the front of my mind was my husband's grandmother Kitty, who didn't talk about the difficulties of birth; instead she said that it was like 'a beautiful flower opening its petals until it is in full bloom'. This is what I concentrated on every time I experienced an intense wave, trusting that all that was happening was my cervix blossoming into this beautiful flower.

Our second midwife on duty walked in around 8 a.m. and we asked if we could be moved to one of the birth-pool rooms. I was feeling very uncomfortable as my waters were continuing to flow; I was walking around wet, and just wanted to sit in some water for a while. You can imagine how incredulous I felt when I was told they were out of use because every one of them had broken thermometers. If I had been told this when I enquired hours earlier, we would have driven to a different hospital.

I had anticipated and prepared for a water birth. So, of course, because we were getting into a heated discussion about why we hadn't been told the birth pools were out of order when we first rang, I stopped being part of what my body was doing and started feeling as if it was being done to me. Suddenly I couldn't cope with the intensity of the contractions – especially as I was once again cheerfully told that I 'hadn't made any progress yet'. I asked if I could have gas and air and was refused. I was so angry with myself for not going with my gut feeling that a home birth would have been fine for me as a first-time mother. In that moment, I hated the midwife; I knew that I had lost my mojo and it was time to call Kicki.

On reflection, my main concern about childbirth (and perhaps this is the same for many women) was the complete lack of control I expected to have. You just have to surrender to what your body is doing, the weird sounds you are making, and the fact that it will take as long as it takes. So the little things you can hold on to that provide some resemblance of choice and control were very important for my wellbeing.

Not long after our emotional discussion with our second midwife, Kicki arrived and immediately sent an email to her contacts in the NHS. Within half an hour, the head midwife came down, apologised and immediately set up a gas and air cylinder (Entonox). Kicki got me up on the bed, leaning over the raised bed head, and helped me get in a better position for opening up my pelvis as I rocked my hips. I was back in control. The next time I let a midwife examine me, I was eight and a half centimetres dilated.

The whole world retreated. I was no longer conscious of who was present, the heavy heat of the room, or the murmurings of my husband and Kicki. I had journeyed far inwards and all my thoughts quietened.

During this time my breathing, my rocking, the note I sighed as I breathed out, my husband's strong hands soothing my back, were all that I was, all that I felt.

Some time passed, and in between administering homeopathic remedies, Kicki insisted that I drink, get up and walk to the bathroom to wee. I did not want to leave my position and remember saying, 'You're a big meanie!' Such maturity from a thirty-eight-year-old! But the walk did speed things up.

It felt like I was having double peaks of waves, and I wasn't sure I had the stamina to continue drug-free. Especially when I found out that my TENS machine only went up to 78 (I thought I had until at least 100 to ramp it up). So I asked Mark to find a midwife, as I wanted some pethidine. While he was looking for a midwife, Kicki quietly helped me concentrate on my breathing and reassured me that she was confident that I was close, and this was as intense as it would get. And then an amazing thing happened. With no pushing, no strain, no added effort on my part, the intensity lessened and my daughter begin to slide through my cervix. I hadn't made any sound besides my breathing note until now, and the sudden change brought forward a soft grunt. Everything fell into place and my labour became effortless. It felt so right ... almost exhilarating.

Our third midwife walked in with a student midwife and Mark. I remember Kicki saying something along the lines of, 'She is involuntarily pushing.' Although I had said in my birth plan that I wanted to give birth on all fours, by now I knew that I wanted to be on my left side. I quickly grabbed my husband by the shirt and pulled him towards me so that I could bury my face in his neck and just breathe in the smell of his skin. As twee as it sounds, gas and air was a pale comparison to the comfort and strength I gained from breathing in the scent of my anchor and soul mate.

The midwife said that they had to move me to the delivery suite and asked me: 'Could you just hop down onto this wheelchair and we can take you through?' In a normal state my response would have been something along the lines of, 'I have something bigger than a rugby ball between my legs, and you want me to delicately hop down and sit on a wheelchair?' Amazingly, I controlled my verbal comeback with a definitive 'No!' Kicki pointed out that my bed had wheels, so asked if I could be wheeled to the delivery room. Great idea.

Once there, Kicki hopped up on the bed and rested my right leg on her shoulder while the midwife took care of the business end. To this day, I wonder at the strength Kicki had, staying in that position for an hour and a half. I could feel Freya moving down with every wave. I didn't have to consciously push; I just breathed her out – it was power personified. I have talked about the battle scars of pregnancy and labour, and to me labour is the ultimate personal battle, where you are the fierce and powerful warrior.

I didn't feel the 'ring of fire' that you sometimes hear the crowning referred to as. This is because Freya came out, Superman-style, with her head and her arm up, so quickly that I tore. I'll be honest; that wasn't my favourite part of the experience. But it happened in an instant, and the midwife used her hands to support my perineum as best she could.

Our beautiful girl was born at 2.24 p.m. on 17th February weighing 7 pounds, 6½ ounces. Because I had had minimal examinations, Kicki estimated that active labour took just under three hours. Freya was immediately placed on my stomach and gave a few short, sweet cries while we waited for the cord to stop pulsating, Mark to cut the cord, and the physiological delivery of the placenta. My own grandmother summed up how awe-inspiring birthing is in these words: 'In that instant, as you hold your newborn for the very first time, you feel you are the queen of the world.'

Many mothers speak of the instant bonding and love flowing through them as they hold their new-borns. As Freya lay on my tummy, I felt a deep respect and an immense responsibility to never take for granted the privilege we had been given in loving and caring for this perfect being lying on me. Kicki took a couple of photos at this time that I will always treasure: one with Mark resting one hand on my head, one hand on his daughter's, his face all scrunched up, crying, a mirror image of his daughter's face. The second photo is of the placenta. Kicki unfurled it, displaying it like the tree of life it is. From a mother's point of view, it is incredible to see just what was created from the cell that split from Freya.

We spent the minimum number of hours in hospital and discharged ourselves that evening. Finally, Mark and I could lie on our own comfortable bed and immerse ourselves in the love of our new family – which included tracing our fingers over every inch of our daughter. Her perfect lips, her neat little fingers, the soft lobes of her ears. Bliss.

Kicki came over several times during the next few weeks, and I am so thankful that she never once showed any signs of being bored at my endless stories of how well Freya's birth had gone, and how grateful we had been to have her there. And how do I feel now about birth? I feel incredibly fortunate that I have been lucky enough to have experienced nurturing and bringing a life into this world. How great it is to be female!

Every woman will embark on her own journey and give birth her own way.

CR80

Chapter 8: Parting Words

The title of this book is *The Secrets of Birth*. I wanted to write it so that I could share with you what I have observed, witnessed and experienced during my time as a mother and as a doula. You might have picked up this book looking for solutions or answers to some very real challenges, or you might have opened it as a curious traveller, just passing through. As you have probably realised by now, this book is not written to solve problems – or, indeed, tell you what to do. My intention was to provide you with tools and information that you can use during what I believe to be some of the greatest experiences a woman can have.

I love and admire women and I'm passionate about supporting them in everything they do. During my years of working with women, not only during pregnancy and birth but also with women attending my doula courses and other projects I'm involved in, I see such courage, determination and adaptability. Most women don't see themselves as having these qualities, and I feel that this can often be traced back to the way they were treated and the way they felt during the birth of their children. I'm not talking about the way they gave birth, but how their emotional wellbeing was cared for and how involved they felt in the decision-making.

I know that giving birth and being a mother are powerful experiences that provide unique opportunities for growth to a woman. Many women do not realise that there are so many factors during the childbearing years that will impact on their behaviour and force changes to take place. For instance, the needs of the baby and the family become the number-one priority for most women, and they may have to find a number of different strategies for managing difficult situations with their children, revealing a hitherto unknown depth of imagination and perseverance.

Often what would make many situations a lot easier is the realisation that it is OK to feel helpless and that, often, we simply need to surrender to what is. Always looking for what to do might not necessarily be the best way forward; sometimes, as soon as we accept the situation as it is, solutions appear. It is easy to become rigid and inflexible when we feel we are losing control or we start feeling exposed or vulnerable. Fear is very influential in triggering behaviour that might make our situation more unbearable and difficult than it has to be. The theme throughout this book has been to explore being more flexible and open to accepting situations as they are, and then look for a way forward. It's not about giving up; it's about giving in to what the present moment brings. Ultimately, it is our mind that translates our experience, and we can choose to become victims or we can look at the experience as an opportunity to change.

I would like to invite women – after experiencing childbirth and mothering – to identify what they discovered about themselves during this process, and apply it to other areas of their lives. As I said before, women do not always see the impact of birth and mothering on their lives, or how they can use the skills and knowledge they gain from these experiences throughout their lives. There are too many women carrying around guilt about things they think they should have done differently and who are beating themselves up for not having had all the information when they made choices about their birth or parenting approaches. I don't want any woman to feel like that!

There is nothing in life that is 100% safe, but when a woman is pregnant, she wants everything to be just that: 100% safe. Going out for a walk, driving, or spending a day at a theme park all carry a certain amount of risk, although this is usually very low. Being pregnant and preparing for birth carries risks too, but no bigger than most things we do each day, in a pregnancy that is without complications. We might not even feel that we are making a choice about remaining safe when we live our lives normally.

I want to see women become aware of the fact that childbirth is statistically over 99% safe (Birthplace in England Collaborative Group, 2011) and that many things that women take for granted and say yes to might not be safe or even always necessary. There is little evidence to ensure the safety of repeated 3D scans, and no study is conclusive enough to say whether inducing labour when the pregnancy goes beyond forty-two weeks actually means a better outcome for the baby. Although the part of the brain that handles critical thinking is somewhat numbed when our brains are full of oxytocin, pregnant women should actively consider all the information they receive with a critical eye.

I took my car for an MOT at KwikFit once, as they offered a free annual service. I had a phone call from the mechanic, i.e. the expert, telling me that I needed to have all my brake pads and discs replaced or my car wouldn't pass the MOT. It was going to cost me a lot of money and I was at a loss. What should I do? Then it occurred to me that perhaps the mechanic was wrong – he had only given me his opinion, not a fact, so I told him to just put the car through the MOT and I'd take my chances. Guess what? It passed!

Yes, I know that having a car MOT'd and giving birth are not the same thing, and a baby is much more precious than a car. However, becoming aware of what you take for granted to be 'the truth' means that you can ask the right questions and look for the research that supports statements made by experts. I invite you to consider getting a second opinion, question anything that is unclear, and ask for evidence to support and back up any medical advice you are given. It is important that birth is safe for both the baby and the woman: however, what's also important is how the woman feels about herself afterwards. A good birth experience doesn't mean everything necessarily goes to plan, but it does mean that the birthing woman feels part of the event and involved in the decisions made about her body and her baby.

I hope that this book has added to your knowledge, and that you now feel that you have more information about childbirth and mothering. In my view, childbirth has become too medicalised and there are too many myths surrounding it. Obstetricians have been allowed to practice based on their peers' opinions and guesses rather than evidence-based information. The power is often taken away from the woman and instead placed within a system that focuses on the prevention of problems and worries about litigation.

There is no other time in a woman's life when she gets a better chance to learn more about herself and who she is. What matters to me is that no woman ever suffers in childbirth or feels guilty as a mother. This has an impact on the baby, the family and society as a whole, which ultimately means an impact on the world. I think that if all women were treated like goddesses during childbirth, there would be a whole bunch of superwomen out there, raising super-powered kids – our future generation. This, for me, is the ultimate goal: if we can get birth right, we could change the world!

Nature doesn't compete with itself; it just is, and it is usually enough. Women need to start believing this too: that they are enough, that they have within themselves what it takes to birth their baby and become a great mother.

Every woman will embark on her own journey and give birth her own way. It is very likely to involve some strong and powerful sensations, and sometimes also pain medication or surgery. She will also find her own ways of being a mother, and mothering is likely to involve guilt, sadness, happiness, elation, frustration, overwhelming love and an array of other emotions. What I am absolutely certain of is that birth and mothering have something extremely valuable to teach a woman about herself – and that is the most important secret of birth.

Birth and mothering have something extremely valuable to teach a woman about herself.

References

Abraham, E., Hendler, T. Shapira-Lichter, I., et al. (2014) Father's brain is sensitive to childcare experiences. *Proceedings of the National Academy of Sciences*, 8 July, III(27), 9792–9797. Available at: doi:10.1073/pnas.1402569111 (accessed 25 September 2017).

Armstrong, J. E. (2002) Breastfeeding and lowering the risk of childhood obesity. *Lancet*, 8 June, 359, 9322, 2003–2004. Available at: http://dx.doi.org/10.1016/S0140-6736(02)08837-2 (accessed 25 September 2017).

Bell, A. F., Erickson, E. N. and Carter, C. S. (2014) Beyond labor: The role of natural and synthetic oxytocin in the transition to motherhood. *Journal of Midwifery & Women's Health*, January/February, 59(1), 35–42. Available at: doi:10.1111/jmwh.12101 (accessed 25 September 2017).

Birthplace in England Collaborative Group (2011) Perinatal and maternal outcomes by planned place of birth for healthy women with low-risk pregnancies: the Birthplace in England national prospective cohort study. *British Medical Journal*, 25 November, 343, d7400. Available at: http://dx.doi.org/10.1136/bmj.d7400 (accessed 25 September 2017).

Birthrights (2013) The Dignity Survey 2013: women's and midwives' experiences of UK maternity care. Birthrights Dignity in Childbirth Forum, October. Available at: http://www.birthrights.org.uk/campaigns/dignity-in-childbirth/dignity-survey/ (accessed 25 September 2017).

Bowlby, J. (1958) The nature of the child's tie to his mother. *International Journal of Psycho-Analysis*, 39, 350–373. Available at: www.psychology.sunysb.edu/attachment/online/nature%20of%20the%20childs%20tie%20bowlby.pdf (accessed 25 September 2017).

Dahlen, H. G., Tracy, S., Tracy, M., et al. (2012) Rates of obstetric intervention among low-risk women giving birth in private and public hospitals in NSW: a population-based descriptive study. *BMJ Open*.

Available at: doi:10.1136/bmjopen-2012-001723 (accessed 25 September 2017).

Dare, M. R., Middleton, P., Crowther, C. A., et al. (2017) Planned early birth versus expectant management (waiting) for pre-labour rupture of membranes at term (37 weeks or more). *The Cochrane Database of Systematic Reviews*. Available at: http://onlinelibrary.wiley.com/doi/10.1002/14651858.CD005302.pub3/pdf (accessed 25 September 2017).

Darmasseelane, K., Hyde, M. J., Santhakumaran, S., et al. (2014) Mode of delivery and offspring body mass index, overweight and obesity in adult life: A systematic review and meta-analysis. *PLOS One*. Available at: http://journals.plos.org/plosone/article?id=10.1371/ journal.pone.0087896 (accessed 25 September 2017).

Devane, D., Lalor, J. G., Daly, S., et al. (2017) Cardiotocography versus intermittent auscultation of fetal heart on admission to labour ward for assessment of fetal wellbeing. *The Cochrane Database of Systematic Reviews*, 26 January, 1. Available at: https://www.ncbi.nlm.nih.gov/pubmed/28125772 (accessed 25 September 2017).

Gaskin, I. M. (2004) Understanding birth and sphincter law. *British Journal of Midwifery*, September, 12, 9. Available at: www.birthlore.com/wp-content/uploads/2012/09/sphincter-law.pdf (accessed 25 September 2017).

Harman, T. (director) (2014) *Microbirth* (motion picture). Available at: http://microbirth.com/ (accessed 25 September 2017).

Hodnett, E. D., Gates, S., Hofmeyr, G. and Sakala, C. (2017) Continuous support for women during childbirth. *The Cochrane Database of Systematic Reviews*. 6 July. Available at: doi:10.1002/14651858.CD003766.pub6 (accessed 25 September 2017).

Jacobson, B., Nyberg, K., Grönbladh, L., et al. (1990) Opiate addiction in adult offspring through possible imprinting after obstetric treatment.

British Medical Journal, 10 November, 301(6760), 1067–1070. Available at: www.ncbi.nlm.nih.gov/pubmed/2249068 (accessed 25 September 2017).

Kitzinger, S. (1999) Obstetric metaphors and marketing. *Birth – Issues in Perinatal Care*. March, 26, 1. Available at: https://www.deepdyve.com/lp/wiley/sheila-kitzinger-s-letter-from-europe-obstetric-metaphors-and-njGGX94e0f (accessed 25 September 2017).

McDonald, S. J., Middleton, P., Dowswell, T. and Morris, P. S. (2013) Effect of timing of umbilical cord clamping of term infants on mother and baby outcomes. *Cochrane Review*. Available at: www.cochrane.org/CD004074/PREG_effect-of-timing-of-umbilical-cord-clamping-of-term-infants-on-mother-and-baby-outcomes (accessed 25 September 2017).

Mendelson, C. (2009) Mini-review: fetal–maternal hormonal signaling in pregnancy and labor. *Molecular Endocrinology*, July, 23(7), 947–954. Available at: doi:10.1210/me.2009-0016 (accessed 25 September 2017).

Middlemiss, W., Granger, D. A., Goldberg, W. A. and Nathans, L. (2011) Asynchrony of mother–infant hypothalamic–pituitary–adrenal axis activity following extinction of infant crying responses induced during the transition to sleep. *Early Human Development*, April 2012, 88(4), 227–232. Available at: doi:10.1016/j.earlhumdev.2011.08.010 (accessed 25 September 2017).

Moore, E. R., Anderson, G. C., Bergman, N. and Dowswell, T. (2012) Early skin-to-skin contact for mothers and their healthy newborn infants. *Cochrane Review*. Available at: www.cochrane.org/CD003519/PREG_early-skin-to-skin-contact-for-mothers-and-their-healthy-newborn-infants (accessed 25 September 2017).

Pascali-Bonaro, D. (director) (2008) *Orgasmic Birth* (motion picture). Available at: https://www.orgasmicbirth.com/products/films-soundtrack/ (accessed 25 September 2017).

Parkington, H. C., Stevenson, J., Tonta, M. A., et al. (2014) Diminished hERG K+ channel activity facilitates strong human labour contractions but is dysregulated in obese women. *Nature Communications*, June, 17(5), Article 4108. Available at: doi:10.1038/ncomms5108 (accessed 25 September 2017).

Postel, T. (2013) Childbirth climax: The revealing of obstetrical orgasm. *Sexologies*, 22(4), e89–e92. Available at: https://www.researchgate.net/publication/259144620_Childbirth_climax_The_revealing_of_obstetrical_orgasm (accessed 25 September 2017).

Prusova, L. C., Churcher, L., Tyler, A. and Lokugamage, A. U. (2014) Royal College of Obstetricians and Gynaecologists guidelines: How evidence-based are they? *Journal of Obstetrics and Gynaecology*, 34(8), 706–711. Available at: doi:**10.3109/01443615.2014.920794** (accessed 25 September 2017).

Public Health England (2012) Ultrasound and infrasound: HPA response to AGNIR report (RCE-14). Available at: https://www.gov.uk/government/publications/ultrasound-and-infrasound-hpa-response-to-agnir-report-rce-14/ (accessed 25 September 2017).

Romano, A. M. (2008) Research summaries for normal birth. *Journal of Perinatal Education*, Spring, 17(2), 54–58. Available at: doi:10.1624/105812408X298408 (accessed 25 September 2017).

Scott, R. (director) (1979) *Alien* (motion picture).

Simkin, P. and Klaus, P. (2004) *When Survivors Give Birth*. Classic Day Publishing.

Smith, J., Platt, F. and Fisk, N. M. (2008) The natural Caesarean: a woman-centred technique. *British Journal of Obstetrics and Gynaecology*, 1037–1042, discussion 1042. Available at: https://www.ncbi.nlm.nih.gov/pmc/articles/PMC2613254/ (accessed 25 September 2017).

'The natural Caesarean: a woman-centred technique' (2011). Available at: https://youtu.be/wdyzAuc3Ff8 (accessed 25 September 2017).

Vardo, J. H., Thornburg, L. L. and Glantz, J. C. (2011) Maternal and neonatal morbidity among nulliparous women undergoing elective induction of labor. *Journal of Reproductive Medicine*, January/February, 56(1–2), 25–30. Available at: www.ncbi.nlm.nih.gov/pubmed/21366123 (accessed 25 September 2017).

Weir, P. (director) (1998) *The Truman Show* (motion picture).

Wickham, S. (2001) Vitamin K: an alternative perspective. *AIMS Journal*, Summer, 13(2). Available at: www.aims.org.uk/Journal/Vol13No2/vitk.htm (accessed 25 September 2017).

Resources

Books

Buckley, S. (2013) *Gentle Birth, Gentle Mothering: A Doctor's Guide to Natural Childbirth and Gentle Early Parenting Choices.* Celestial Arts.

Graves, K. (2012) *The Hypnobirthing Book: An Inspirational Guide for a Calm, Confident, Natural Birth.* Katharine Publishing.

Schiller, R. (2014) *All That Matters: Women's Rights in Childbirth.* Guardian Shorts.

Sundin, J. (2008) *Birth Skills: Proven Pain-management Techniques for your Labour and Birth.* Vermilion.

Websites

The Secrets of Birth – www.thesecretsofbirth.com

BirthBliss Doula Services – www.birthbliss.co.uk

BirthBliss Academy – www.birthblissacademy.com

Doula UK – www.doula.org.uk

AIMS (Association of Improvements in the Maternity Services) – www.aims.org.uk

Birthrights – www.birthrights.org.uk

NICE (National Institute for Health and Care Excellence) – www.nice.org.uk

NCT – www.nct.org.uk

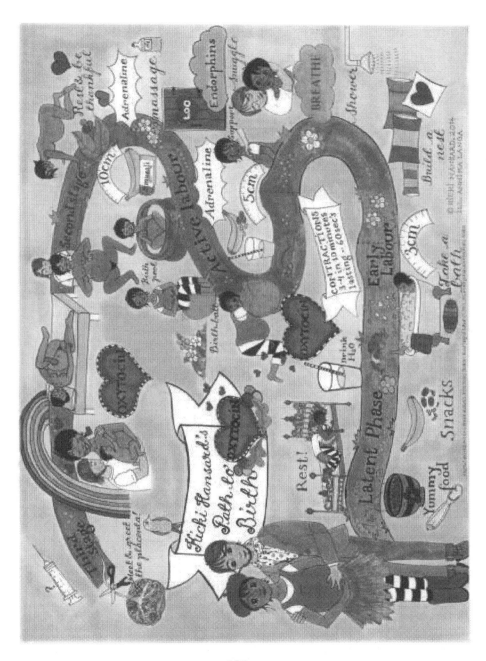

On-line Antenatal Programme

Your Birth - Your Way: The complete online antenatal programme

https://courses.kickihansard.com/p/your-birth-your-way

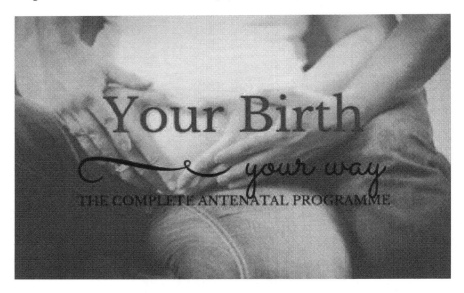

A six week online antenatal programme educating, inspiring and
supporting women as they prepare for the birth of their baby and beyond
- all from the comfort of their own home, anywhere in the world!

Acknowledgements

Thank you to all the women and families that I have had the pleasure to work with, and who have let me into their lives during a time which is so rich in opportunities to learn. I will be forever grateful for their contribution towards my own personal growth and this book.

Thank you to my parents, Maj-Lis and Egon, my sister Karin and brother Andreas, my extended family and all my friends for shaping me into the person I am and for loving me unconditionally.

Thank you to Siobhan and Nicola for always believing in me.

Thank you to Maggie, who came into my life at precisely the moment when I needed her insight and honest feedback.

Thank you to my gorgeous husband, Lance, for always believing in me and for being my mountain and my energiser.

Afterword

If you enjoyed *The Secrets of Birth*, would you be willing to take a minute to write a review on Amazon? Even a short review helps, and it would really mean a lot to me.

If someone you care about is expecting a baby or has just become a parent, please send them a copy of this book. Whether you gift it to them on Amazon or send them your copy makes no difference to me.

If you'd like to order copies of this book for your company, school or group of friends, please email info@thesecretsofbirth.com

Finally, if you'd like to contribute with your very own secrets of birth and parenthood, please visit www.thesecretsofbirth.com to submit your story. Together we can create a place where women can gather and share their stories to support and nurture each other.

Wishing you all the best on your journey!

Kichi x

About the author

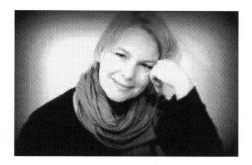

Kicki Hansard is a certified birth and postnatal doula with experience in all aspects of pregnancy, childbirth and parenting. Since 2002, she has been preparing couples for the arrival of their baby, and has supported many of them through the birth and postnatal period. She has been working as a doula course facilitator since 2006, and runs the BirthBliss Aspiring Doula Foundation course. Kicki was also awarded the *Pregnancy & Birth* Magazine and Doula UK award of 'Doula of the Year' in 2009.

Kicki believes that birth is a truly normal, and at the same time, deeply profound event that is optimised by personalised support, defined birth goals with flexibility built in, and solid education. Her goals are to instil confidence along with accurate information, equipping women and families for the work of labour, birth and the postnatal period, and to understand each family's unique needs and birth goals.

Kicki has trained with the 'grandmothers of doulas', Penny Simkin and Phyllis Klaus, in San Diego as a 'When Survivors Give Birth' educator, and has produced 'Kicki Hansard's Path to Birth', an educational tool for birth preparation.

Born in Swedish Lapland, the magical land of the midnight sun and the Northern Lights, Kicki moved to the UK in 1990. She is married with two teenage daughters.

Printed in Great Britain
by Amazon